Understanding Lung Sounds

Third Edition

Understanding Lung Sounds

Steven Lehrer, M.D.

Staff Physician
Veterans Affairs Medical Center
Bronx, New York;
Associate Clinical Professor
Mount Sinai School of Medicine
New York, New York

SAUNDERS

An Imprint of Elsevier

SAUNDERS
An Imprint of Elsevier
The Curtis Center
Independence Square West
Philadelphia, PA 19106

NOTICE

Health care is an ever-changing field. Standard safety precautions must be followed, but as new research and clinical experience broaden our knowledge, changes in treatment and drug therapy may become necessary or appropriate. Readers are advised to check the most current product information provided by the manufacturer of each drug to be administered to verify the recommended dose, the method and duration of administration, and contraindications. It is the responsibility of the licensed prescriber, relying on experience and knowledge of the patient, to determine dosages and the best treatment for each individual patient. Neither the publisher nor the editor assumes any liability for any injury and/or damage to persons or property arising from this publication.

Library of Congress Cataloging-in-Publication Data

Lehrer, Steven.
    Understanding lung sounds / Steven Lehrer.—3rd ed.
        p. ; cm.
    Includes bibliographical references and index.
    ISBN-13: 978-1-4160-6838-9
        1. Auscultation. 2. Lungs—Sounds. 3. Lungs—Examination. I. Title.
    [DNLM: 1. Auscultation. 2. Respiratory Sounds—Diagnosis. WF 141 L524u 2002]
    RC734.A94 L43 2002
    616.2′407544—dc21

                                                                    2001057648

Vice President and Publishing Director: Sally Schrefer
Executive Editor: Robin Carter
Managing Editor: Lee Henderson
Publishing Services Manager: Deborah L. Vogel
Project Manager: Deon Lee
Design Manager: Bill Drone
Cover Designer: Sheilah Barrett

UNDERSTANDING LUNG SOUNDS

ISBN-13: 978-1-4160-6838-9

Printed in the United States of America.

Last digit is the print number: 9   8   7   6   5   4   3   2   GW/MVY

Foreword

Physicians have been listening to lung sounds since several centuries before Christ; witness the succussion splash of hydropneumothorax, which is attributed to Hippocrates. In 1816 Laennec's substitution of the stethoscope for direct application of the ear to the chest ushered in a Golden Age. The phenomenology of abnormal lung sounds was brought to bear on the diagnosis of lung cavities, consolidation, emphysema, and pleural effusions. The Golden Age lasted out the century. Although the importance of stethoscopy in the clinical armamentarium continues to this day, as indicated in this book, the method was partially eclipsed by the advent of the x-ray in 1895, followed by the derivative methods of pulmonary arteriography in the 1950s and CT scanning in the 1970s. Indeed, the eclipse has probably gone too far, because the availability and ease of use of the stethoscope are hard to beat. Thus Dr. Lehrer's book is an important one.

In parallel with the description of the phenomena of lung sounds has been the science of lung sounds. Correlations with the findings of autopsy (Laennec himself initiated this approach) and later correlations with the radiographic findings constituted the main basis of that science, but some studies of the physics of lung sounds date back into the nineteenth century. More recent physical studies include the analyses I made by the method of sound spectrography in the 1950s. The physics of lung sounds continues to absorb the interest of a small but avid group of clinical scientists. Indeed, the Eighth International Conference on Lung Sounds was held here at Johns Hopkins, assembling aficionados from many countries to review their work in this field.

It is the art and science of lung sounds that Steve Lehrer brings together in this useful book on a persistently important part of our clinical armamentarium.

VICTOR A. McKUSICK, M.D.
William Osler Professor and Director,
Department of Medicine,
Johns Hopkins University School of Medicine;
Physician-in-Chief,
Johns Hopkins Hospital,
Baltimore, Maryland

v

Preface

Since antiquity, physicians have examined the chest for signs of disease. Some physical diagnostic signs that are recognized today were first noted by the ancient Greeks. In the eighteenth century percussion techniques were added to the diagnostic repertoire, and in the nineteenth century auscultation was added. For many years, these methods, along with a carefully elicited history, were the only tools available to diagnose chest diseases.

The situation changed dramatically in 1895 with the discovery of x-rays. Suddenly, many chest structures could be observed, as through a window. Diagnosis became considerably more refined and simple to accomplish; all one needed to do was to inspect the x-ray film. The teaching of physical diagnosis of the chest, especially auscultation and the recognition of normal and abnormal breath sounds, received little attention except from chest specialists.

In the past few years, however, interest in breath sounds has been growing. Breath sound analytic techniques, drawing on modern electronic and acoustic advances, have become increasingly sophisticated. Some researchers hope eventually to construct a computerized electronic device able to "listen" to the chest and then produce a data printout of information that can now be obtained only with multiple pulmonary function tests.

The purpose of this book is to teach elementary chest diagnosis and, above all, how to listen to breath sounds. Much new information on the significance of normal and abnormal breath sounds can be found here. In addition, the latest research findings are presented, along with the most significant data, often in graphic form, from each investigator's work. To help the beginning student, some concepts from anatomy, physiology, and pathology are presented; however, this material is not intended to be a complete treatise on the lung. It is only meant to provide enough background information to elucidate the remaining material. Full, detailed discussions of anatomy, physiology, and pathology may be found in the works listed in the bibliography for Chapter 1.

Numerous advances in the study of lung sounds have occurred since the first edition of *Understanding Lung Sounds* was published. There has been progress in lung sound analysis with the advent of a computer method, fast Fourier transformation. At least one new diagnostic sign has been described: poor breath sounds with good voice sounds in bronchial stenosis. Investigators have done comparative analyses of adult and infant lung sounds, noting especially the frequency differences. And some anesthesiologists are now analyzing lung sounds to ensure proper placement of endotracheal tubes. These and other areas of lung sounds research are described in this third edition.

I am grateful to many individuals for the help they gave me while I was writing this book. Dr. David W. Cugell, Dr. Earle B. Weiss, the American College of Chest Physicians, Dr. A. R. Nath, Dr. Steve S. Kraman, Dr. Peter Krumpe, Dr. Roy Donnerberg, Dr. Rand David, and Dr. Marilyn Orenstein provided sounds for the CD accompanying this volume. Gary Hilt helped with the recording of sounds. Margaret Kinney, Kathleen O'Hogan, and Loyola Salva, of the Bronx VA Hospital Medical Library, found many articles for me. Katherine Pitcoff, Frances T. Mues, Anna Congdon, and Betty Gittens, all formerly of the W.B. Saunders Company, provided much invaluable editorial guidance. Dr. David W. Cugell, Dr. Steve S. Kraman, and Dr. Marvin Lesser reviewed the entire manuscript and made many helpful suggestions. Edward M. Jones prepared the original illustrations. Gloria Spevacek, of the Bronx VA Hospital Medical Media Production Service, obtained some of the reference material for me. Blandine Triestman of W.B. Saunders Company was a constant source of support and encouragement.

A final word is in order about the title of this book. The sounds of breathing may be described by three synonymous terms: *lung sounds, breath sounds,* and *respiratory sounds. Lung sounds* is the term often used by researchers. *Breath sounds* is the term frequently employed by physicians, nurses, and respiratory therapists involved in direct patient care. *Respiratory sounds* is the index term used for classification in the *Index Medicus,* which lists all articles on the subject under this one heading. In the following chapters, the three terms will be used interchangeably.

STEVEN LEHRER, M.D.

Contents

Contents of Companion Audio CD

Track 1. Introduction.

Track 2. Normal vesicular breath sounds. These sounds are heard over most of the peripheral parts of the lung.

Track 3. Bronchial breath sounds. These sounds are present normally only over the manubrium.

Track 4. Bronchial breath sounds and audible heart sounds over the chest of a patient with pneumonia.

Track 5. Bronchovesicular breath sounds. The expiratory and inspiratory phases are about equal in length.

Track 6. Tracheal breath sounds. These sounds, not usually auscultated, are present over the extrathoracic portion of the trachea.

Track 7. Breath sounds over a lung cavity (amphorous breath sounds). Expiration is equal in length to inspiration but lower in pitch.

Track 8. High-pitched crackles. These short, explosive, nonmusical sounds are also called *fine crackles*.

Track 9. Low-pitched crackles. These sounds are also called *coarse crackles*.

Track 10. Early inspiratory crackles. These crackles are characteristic of severe airway obstruction.

Track 11. Late inspiratory crackles. These crackles are associated with restrictive pulmonary disease.

Track 12. Death rattle (crackles over mouth). These sounds result from an accumulation of secretions in the airway.

Track 13. Wheezing. A *wheeze* is a musical pulmonary sound. High-pitched wheeze. This sound is sometimes called a *sibilant rhonchus*.

Track 14. Low-pitched wheeze. This sound is sometimes called a *sonorous rhonchus*.

Track 15. Monophonic wheeze. This wheeze is made up of a single musical note.

Track 16. Polyphonic wheeze. This wheeze is composed of several dissonant notes, beginning and ending at the same time.

Track 17. Stridor. This is a particularly loud musical sound of constant pitch, resulting from obstruction of a central airway.

Track 18. Pleural friction rub. This sound resembles the noise made by leather sliding on leather.

Chapter 1

Anatomy, Physiology, and Pathophysiology Review

The purpose of the lung is gas exchange. Its most important function is to allow oxygen to move from the air into the systemic venous blood to meet the metabolic needs of the cells; the lung then allows carbon dioxide, a waste product of cellular metabolism, to move out. This function is accomplished through a series of complex processes. Contraction of the inspiratory muscles results in flow of air through the trachea and bronchi into the alveoli of the lung. Here, alveolar air and pulmonary capillary blood, though separated by an ultrathin alveolar-capillary membrane, come into very close contact. Oxygen diffuses across the alveolar-capillary membrane into the blood while carbon dioxide passes in the opposite direction.

ANATOMY

The lungs are cone-shaped organs that completely fill the pleural spaces. The right lung is divided by fissures into an upper, middle, and lower lobe. The left lung is divided into an upper and lower lobe. Air moves into and out of the lungs through the airways, which are subdivided into two components from a functional point of view: (1) the conducting airways, often called the *tracheobronchial tree,* consisting of the trachea, the bronchi, and the bronchioles; and (2) the terminal respiratory units (sometimes called the *acini*) (Figure 1-1). The conducting airways function chiefly to conduct gas into and out of the terminal respiratory units, where the actual gas exchange takes place.

Conducting Airways

Air enters the gas-exchanging units of the lung by way of the nose or mouth and then passes through the larynx and tracheobronchial system. The upper air passages filter, humidify, and adjust the temperature of inspired air.

1

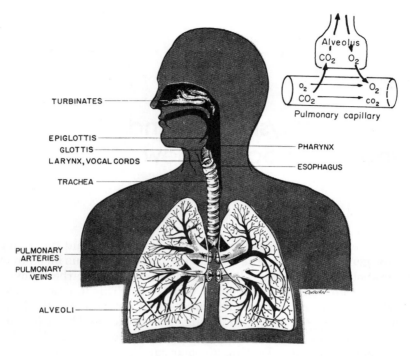

FIGURE 1-1. The respiratory passages. (From Guyton AC, Hall JE: *Textbook of medical physiology,* ed 10, Philadelphia, 2000, WB Saunders.)

Trachea

The extrathoracic portion of the trachea lies in the midline of the anterior part of the neck. After entering the thorax, the trachea deviates slightly to the right. The trachea is supported by horseshoe-shaped rings of cartilage, connected posteriorly by a pliable membrane. During coughing, the increased pressure within the thorax pushes the membrane into the space between the arms of the cartilages, narrowing the lumen significantly. Consequently, velocity of airflow increases, creating a shearing force that dislodges material lying on the mucosal surface.

The trachea divides into the right and left main bronchi at the carina. The right bronchus leaves the bifurcation at less of an angle than does the left bronchus; for this reason, aspirated fluids are more prone to enter the right lung. Because the right-sided displacement of the trachea within the thorax carries it away from the left lung and closer to the right, the left main bronchus is longer (5 cm) than the right (3 cm).

The bronchi are divided into lobar and segmental branches (Figure 1-2). Familiarity with these divisions, especially the bronchopulmonary segments, is important because some lung diseases are characteristically found within particular segments. For example, pulmonary tuberculosis

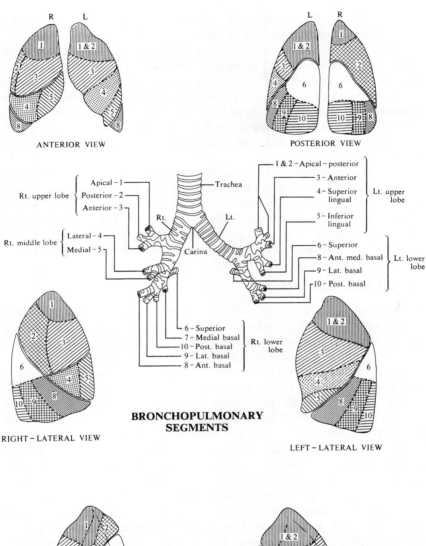

BRONCHOPULMONARY SEGMENTS

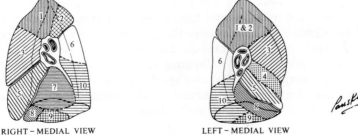

FIGURE 1-2. The trachea and the bronchopulmonary segments. (From Pansky B, House EL: *Review of gross anatomy,* ed 3, New York, 1975, Macmillan Publishing.)

is most likely to affect the apical and posterior upper lobe segments or the superior segment of the lower lobes.

A bronchopulmonary segment is a wedge of lung tissue that is supplied by a single segmental bronchus and its corresponding pulmonary artery. The venous drainage of the segments is variable, with a vein often draining more than one segment. Each segment functions as a relatively independent unit, although there is some collateral circulation and ventilation between adjacent segments. The segments are irregular in shape and variable in size and are separated by thin, incomplete connective tissue barriers.

The bronchi subdivide into smaller and smaller passages, referred to as generations. The last and smallest branches, from which the terminal respiratory units originate, are called *terminal bronchioles*. Near the hilum of the lung, the terminal bronchioles may be reached with only 10 bronchial branchings; more than 25 branchings may be necessary to reach the terminal bronchioles in the most peripheral basal parts of the lung.

Terminal Respiratory Units

The terminal bronchioles are joined to the terminal respiratory units, also known as the lung parenchyma; here, gas exchange takes place. A group of three to five terminal bronchioles, each with its appended terminal respiratory unit, is usually called a *pulmonary lobule.*

Terminal respiratory units, sometimes called *acini* or *primary lobules,* have a characteristically variable branching pattern. There are usually two to five orders of respiratory bronchioles, the last of which leads to two to five orders of alveolar ducts. Each alveolar duct leads to 10 to 16 alveoli (Figure 1-3). An average adult has 300 million alveoli, but this figure is highly variable, depending on age and body size. Because 90% of the total alveolar surface is covered with pulmonary capillaries, the alveolar capillary surface available for gas exchange is 60 to 70 m^2 in the normal adult (1 m^2 per kilogram of body weight).

Gas in the alveoli does not contact the alveolar epithelium directly; instead, the surface is covered by a layer of fluid containing a substance called *surfactant,* which imparts the lowest surface tension of any biologic material ever tested. Low surface tension at this location is important; it keeps alveoli from collapsing. When surfactant is deficient, as in the neonatal respiratory distress syndrome, atelectasis and severe mechanical disturbances occur. Surfactant is a phospholipid that is secreted by special cells of the alveolar epithelium.

Chest Wall

The thorax, that part of the body between the neck and abdomen, is encased by a bony framework of ribs shaped like a truncated cone and lined

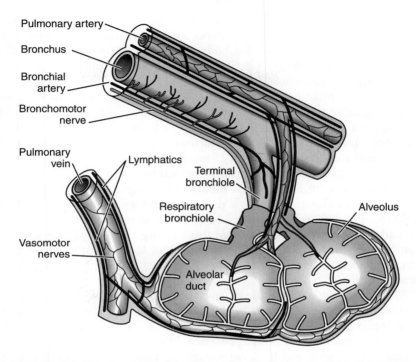

FIGURE 1-3. Structure of the lung. (From Staub NC: *Hum Pathol* 1:419, 1970.)

by the pleura, a fibrous membrane. Between the ribs lie two bands of muscles, the external and internal intercostals. The external intercostal muscles extend from the articulations between the ribs and vertebral bodies to the origins of the costal cartilages. The internal intercostals extend from the sternum to the angles of the ribs. Normal inspiratory breathing at rest is performed by contraction of the muscles of inspiration—the diaphragm and external intercostals; normal expiration is passive and requires no muscular effort. However, when increased amounts of air are necessary, expiration in normal persons becomes active; accessory muscles of respiration in the neck—sternocleidomastoids and scalene—as well as abdominal muscles—rectus, external and internal obliques, and transversus abdominis—are utilized to augment the rate and depth of breathing. Patients with certain lung diseases, such as asthma and emphysema, often need to use expiratory muscles and accessory muscles to maintain adequate ventilation at rest.

PHYSIOLOGY

The process of respiration can be divided into three major mechanistic events: (1) pulmonary ventilation—the inflow and outflow of air between the atmosphere and lung alveoli, (2) diffusion of oxygen and carbon dioxide between the alveoli and the blood, and (3) transport of oxygen and carbon dioxide in the blood and body fluids to and from the cells. Only those aspects of pulmonary ventilation that are most pertinent to an understanding of breath sounds are discussed here.

During inspiration at rest, the intraalveolar pressure becomes slightly negative with respect to atmospheric pressure, normally slightly less than -1 mm Hg, and this causes air to flow inward through the respiratory passageways. During normal expiration at rest, the intraalveolar pressure rises to slightly less than $+1$ mm Hg, causing air to flow outward through the respiratory passageways.

The lungs have a continual elastic tendency to collapse and recoil away from the chest wall. Two different factors cause this tendency: (1) elastic fibers throughout the lung that are stretched during inflation and (2) surface tension of the fluid lining the alveoli, which tends to pull them closed. Without the presence of the previously mentioned surfactant to reduce this surface tension, lung expansion would be extremely difficult.

The compliance of the lungs and thorax is expressed as the volume increase in the lungs for each unit increase in transpulmonary pressure. The compliance of the normal lungs and thorax combined is 0.08 to 0.10 L per centimeter of water pressure. In other words, when the alveolar pressure is increased by 1 cm water, the lungs expand 80 to 100 ml.

The lungs alone, when removed from the chest, are almost twice as distensible as the lungs and thorax together because the thoracic cage must also be stretched when the lungs are expanded within it. Thus the muscles of inspiration use energy both to expand the lungs and to expand the thoracic cage around the lungs. Many pathologic conditions affecting the lung cause decreased compliance. These include deformities of the thoracic cage, such as kyphosis or scoliosis, fibrosis, and interstitial fibrosis.

FIGURE 1-4. Graphic representation of the two different types of work accomplished during inspiration: (1) compliance work, the largest fraction, represented by the trapezoid OAECDO and (2) airway and tissue resistance work, represented by the hatched area ABCEA. *FRC,* Functional residual capacity. (From West JB: *Respiratory physiology—the essentials,* ed 2, Baltimore, 1979, Williams & Wilkins.)

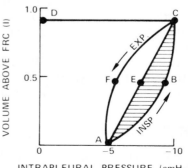

As has been mentioned, during ordinary quiet breathing, muscle contraction occurs only during inspiration; expiration is entirely passive, resulting from elastic recoil of the lung and thorax. The work of inspiration can be divided into two fractions: (1) compliance work, necessary to expand the lung against its elastic forces; and (2) airway and tissue resistance work, needed to overcome the viscosity of lung, chest wall structures, and airway resistance during movement of air into the lungs. These two types of work are illustrated graphically in Figure 1-4. As can be seen, during normal quiet breathing, most of the work done by the respiratory muscles is done merely to expand the lungs (compliance work). But during very heavy breathing, when air must flow through the airways at high velocity, the greatest proportion of the work goes to overcome airway resistance. During normal quiet breathing, only 2% to 3% of the total body energy requirement, measured by oxygen consumption, is needed for pulmonary ventilation; but in the presence of some severe pulmonary diseases such as asthma and emphysema, a third or more of total body energy must be expended for the same purpose.

A simple technique for recording the volume movement of air into and out of the lungs is called *spirometry*. A typical spirometer consists of a drum inverted over a chamber of water, with the drum counterbalanced by a weight (Figure 1-5). The drum contains a breathing mixture of gases, usually air or oxygen; the mouth is connected to the gas chamber by a tube and mouthpiece. When the subject breathes in and out of the mouthpiece, the drum rises and falls, and a recording is made on a moving sheet of paper.

Figure 1-6 is a diagram demonstrating changes in lung volume under different conditions of breathing. In this diagram, air in the lungs has

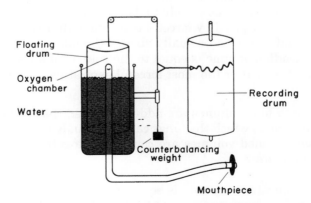

Floating drum

Oxygen chamber

Water

Recording drum

Counterbalancing weight

Mouthpiece

FIGURE 1-5. A spirometer. (From Guyton AC, Hall JE: *Textbook of medical physiology,* ed 10, Philadelphia, 2000, WB Saunders.)

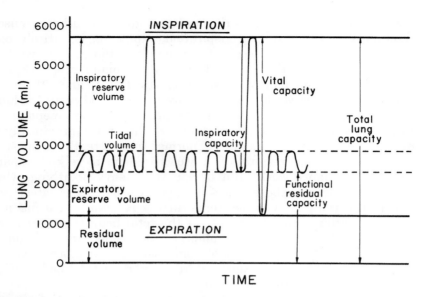

FIGURE 1-6. Diagram showing respiratory excursions during normal breathing and during maximal inspiration and maximal expiration. (From Guyton AC, Hall JE: *Textbook of medical physiology,* ed 10, Philadelphia, 2000, WB Saunders.)

been subdivided into four different volumes and four different capacities (predicted values depend on age, sex, and height).

1. The tidal volume is equal to the volume of air inspired or expired with each normal breath, usually about 500 ml.
2. The inspiratory reserve volume is equal to the extra volume of air that can be inspired over and beyond the normal tidal volume, usually about 3000 ml.
3. The expiratory reserve volume is equal to the amount of air that can still be expired by forceful expiration after the end of a normal tidal expiration, usually about 1100 ml.
4. The residual volume is equal to the volume of air still remaining in the lungs after the most forceful expiration, usually about 1200 ml.

When these four volumes are added together, they are equal to the maximum volume to which the lungs can be expanded. When two or more of the aforementioned volumes are considered together, they are called *pulmonary capacities.*

1. The inspiratory capacity is equal to the tidal volume plus inspiratory reserve volume, about 3500 ml. This is the amount of air that a subject can breathe beginning at the normal expiratory level and distending the lungs maximally.

2. The functional residual capacity is equal to the expiratory reserve volume plus residual volume, about 2300 ml. This is the amount of air remaining in the lungs at the end of normal expiration.
3. The vital capacity is equal to inspiratory reserve volume plus tidal volume plus expiratory reserve volume, about 4600 ml. This is the maximum amount of air that a subject can expel from the lungs after they are first filled to the maximum extent and then expired to the maximum extent.
4. The total lung capacity is equal to the maximum volume to which the lungs can be expanded with the greatest possible inspiratory effort, about 5800 ml (this includes vital capacity and residual volume).

When all inspiratory muscles are completely relaxed, the lungs return to a resting state called the *resting expiratory level*. The volume of air in the lungs is then equal to the functional residual capacity, about 2300 ml in the young adult.

Each of the pulmonary volumes and capacities has a specific significance. Moreover, each changes with the position of the body; most decrease when the subject lies down and increase when the subject stands up. Two factors account for this change: (1) the abdominal contents press upward against the diaphragm in the lying position, and (2) pulmonary blood volume increases in the lying position. Both of these changes decrease the space available for pulmonary air.

The residual volume, the air that cannot be removed from the lungs even by forceful expiration, furnishes air in the alveoli to aerate the blood, even between breaths. Were there no residual volume, the concentrations of oxygen and carbon dioxide in the blood would rise and fall markedly with each breath.

Any of the following abnormalities tends to diminish the vital capacity:

1. *Paralysis of the respiratory muscles.* This often occurs after spinal cord injuries or poliomyelitis and can decrease vital capacity to 1000 to 500 ml.
2. *Diminished pulmonary compliance ("stiff lungs").* Tuberculosis, lung cancer, and pulmonary fibrosis all can reduce pulmonary compliance and thereby decrease vital capacity.
3. *Pulmonary vascular congestion.* In left-sided heart failure or any other condition causing pulmonary vascular congestion and edema, vital capacity is reduced because excess fluid in the lungs decreases compliance.

Another very important measurement of ventilatory function is the *maximum expiratory flow rate*. When a person expires with progressively increasing force, the expiratory airflow rate reaches a maximum, despite further increase in expiratory force. This effect can be understood by referring to Figure 1-7, *A*. When pressure is applied to the lungs by chest cage compression, the same amount of pressure is applied to the exterior of both the alveoli and the respiratory passages, as indicated by the arrows. Consequently, not only is the pressure increased in the alveoli to force air to the exterior, but also the terminal bronchioles are collapsed at the same time, increasing airway resistance. Beyond a certain point, these two effects have equal but opposite results on airflow.

Figure 1-7, *B* illustrates this phenomenon. The plotted curve is the expiratory flow achieved by a normal subject who first inhales as much air as possible and then expires with maximum effort until he can expire no further. Note that an expiratory airflow of over 400 L/min is rapidly reached. However, no matter how much additional effort is exerted, this is the maximum expiratory flow that can be achieved.

Note also that as lung volume decreases, maximum expiratory flow decreases, principally because in the enlarged lung, the bronchi are held open partially by elastic pull on their exteriors by structural elements of the lung. However, as the lung becomes smaller, these structures are relaxed, and the bronchi collapse more easily.

Maximum expiratory flow–volume curves are often recorded in the pulmonary function laboratory to determine ventilatory abnormalities. In restrictive disease (constricted lungs), both total lung capacity (TLC)

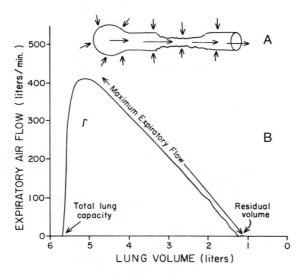

FIGURE 1-7. A, Collapse of the respiratory passageway during maximal expiratory effort; this effect limits the expiratory flow rate. **B,** Effect of lung volume on the maximal expiratory airflow; note the decreasing maximal expiratory airflow as the lung volume becomes smaller. (From Guyton AC, Hall JE: *Textbook of medical physiology,* ed 10, Philadelphia, 2000, WB Saunders.)

and residual volume (RV) are diminished. In addition, because the lung cannot expand to its normal volume, even with the greatest expiratory effort, the maximal expiratory flow rate cannot rise to normal. Among the restrictive lung diseases are advanced tuberculosis and silicosis; diffuse interstitial pulmonary fibrosis of unknown etiology; kyphosis and scoliosis, which constrict the chest cage; drug-induced fibrotic reactions; and fibrosis secondary to chemical or physical injury.

In the presence of airway obstruction, expiration is usually much more difficult than inspiration because the expiratory closing tendency of the airways is greatly increased, whereas the negative intrapleural pressure of inspiration actually "pulls" the airways open. Consequently, air tends to enter the lung easily, where it becomes trapped. Moreover, because of partial obstruction of many airways and because they collapse more easily than normal airways, maximum expiratory flow is significantly diminished. Severe airway obstruction occurs in asthma, chronic bronchitis, bronchiectasis, and emphysema.

A simple, useful test of airway obstruction is the *forced expiratory vital capacity (FVC)*. Recordings of FVC, made on a spirometer, are shown in Figure 1-8, *A,* for a subject with normal lungs, and in Figure 1-8, *B,* for a subject with respiratory obstruction. To obtain the recording, the examiner asks the subject to inspire maximally to total lung capacity, then to exhale into the spirometer with maximum expiratory effort as rapidly and completely as possible. The total excursion of the record represents the FVC, as illustrated in the figure.

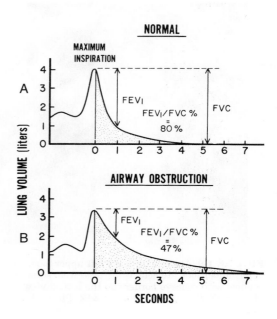

FIGURE 1-8. Spirometer recordings made during a forced vital capacity test *(FVC)* in a normal subject **(A),** and in a subject with airway obstruction **(B).** *FEV₁,*Forced expiratory volume during the first second. (From Guyton AC, Hall JE: *Textbook of medical physiology,* ed 10, Philadelphia, 2000, WB Saunders.)

In normal lungs and lungs with obstructed airways, the FVCs may be equal, but often they are not, due in part to air trapping. In addition, there is a marked difference in the flow rate at which the subjects can expire, especially within the first second. This forced expiratory volume during the first second (FEV_1) is recorded and used for comparison between normal and abnormal. In a normal subject, the FVC expired in the first second (FEV_1/ FVC%) is about 80%. However, in the subject with airway obstruction shown in Figure 1-8, *B,* this value has decreased to only 47%. In severe airway obstruction, often seen in acute asthma, the value can decrease to less than 20%.

The most important factor in the entire ventilatory process is the rate at which the air is renewed each minute by atmospheric air in the gas-exchange area of the lungs—the alveoli, the alveolar sacs, the alveolar ducts, and the respiratory bronchioles; this process is called *alveolar ventilation.* Obviously, considerably less gas flows into the alveoli than flows into the lungs because a large portion of the inspired air goes to fill respiratory passageways, the membranes of which are incapable of significant gaseous exchange with the blood. This air is referred to as *dead-space air.* No breath sounds are believed to be produced by alveolar ventilation.

The mechanisms that produce abnormal breath sounds may be best comprehended with an understanding of the major pathologic processes and alterations that can occur in the lung. A brief description of these is presented in the following section.

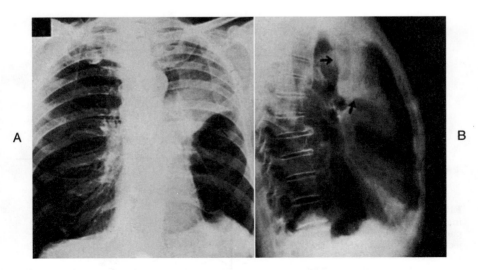

A

B

FIGURE 1-9. Atelectasis of the left upper lobe. Posteroanterior **(A)** and lateral **(B)** views of left upper lobe atelectasis *(arrows)* from squamous cell carcinoma. The triangular shadow with concave borders on the lateral view is characteristic. (From Hinshaw HC, Murray JF: *Diseases of the chest,* ed 4, Philadelphia, 1980, WB Saunders.)

PATHOLOGY
Atelectasis

Atelectasis is a condition in which a portion of the lungs is unexpanded. A whole lung, a lobe, or only small segments within a lobe may be involved. Congenital atelectasis is failure of the lungs to expand fully in the neonatal period. Functional atelectasis results from incomplete inflation of the lungs during quiet breathing.

Acquired atelectasis is either obstructive or compressive. Obstructive atelectasis results from an obstruction of the trachea or bronchi; it may be caused by aspiration of a foreign body, a tumor mass occluding the bronchus, or exudate. A large area of atelectasis, often called *massive collapse,* may cause the heart to be displaced to the affected side. Compressive atelectasis results from compression of the lung by fluid or air in the pleural or pericardial space, a large intrathoracic tumor (Figure 1-9), or elevation of the diaphragm. When the atelectatic lung expands, crackles are heard through the stethoscope because of the sudden opening of airways (see Chapter 5).

Emphysema

Emphysema is an abnormal enlargement of the air spaces accompanied by destruction of the alveolar walls; these changes produce considerable increase in the volume of the lungs (Figure 1-10). Emphy-

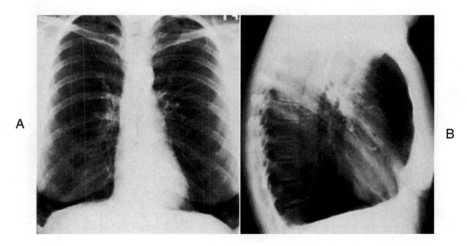

FIGURE 1-10. Roentgenographic findings in emphysema. Posteroanterior **(A)**and lateral **(B)** chest x-rays of a 62-year-old woman with advanced chronic obstructive pulmonary disease, mainly emphysema, showing low flattened diaphragms, large retrosternal air space, vertically oriented heart, and hyperlucent lung fields. (From Hinshaw HC, Murray JF: *Diseases of the chest,* ed 4, Philadelphia, 1980, WB Saunders.)

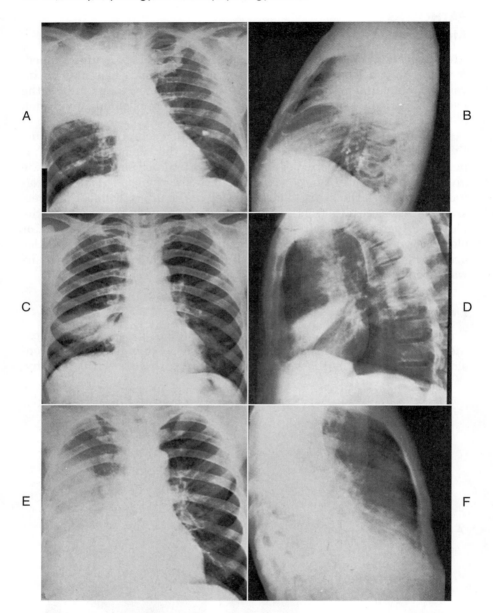

FIGURE 1-11. Consolidation in three cases of verified pneumococcal pneumonia involving the right upper lobe (**A** and **B**), the right middle lobe (**C** and **D**), and the right lower lobe (**E** and **F**). (From Hinshaw HC, Murray JF: *Diseases of the chest,* ed 4, Philadelphia, 1980, WB Saunders.)

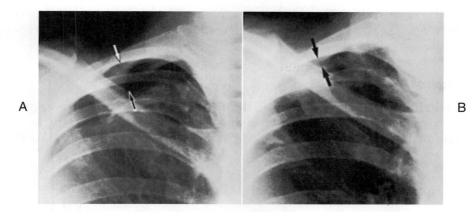

FIGURE 1-12. Small pneumothorax. Detailed views of right upper lung and chest wall. Note that the air gap *(arrows)* is wider and more apparent in expiration **(A)** than in inspiration **(B).** (From Hinshaw HC, Murray JF: *Diseases of the chest,* ed 4, Philadelphia, 1980, WB Saunders.)

sema usually requires many years to develop into the advanced stages characterized by shortness of breath and barrel chest. The physical findings include increase in anteroposterior diameter of the chest, fixation of the chest with the ribs in a more nearly horizontal plane, and use of the accessory muscles of respiration. Diminished breath sounds are heard through the stethoscope (see Chapter 5). In the Western world, cigarette smoking is virtually the only cause of emphysema. The single significant exception is α_1-antitrypsin deficiency, an enzyme deficiency, which is rare.

Consolidation

Consolidation, which is a solidifying of lung tissue because of the presence of large amounts of fluid, is a hallmark of pneumonia. Bronchial breath sounds, egophony, whispered pectoriloquy, and bronchophony are heard over a consolidated lung (Figure 1-11) (see Chapter 5).

Pneumothorax

Pneumothorax occurs when air enters the pleural space, permitting partial or total collapse of a lung, often in otherwise normal young people. Air escapes into the pleural cavity because of rupture of a distended bleb on the surface of the lung. Pneumothorax may also result from laceration of the lung caused by a fractured rib, a puncture wound, or tuberculosis (Figure 1-12). Breath sounds will be absent over one side of the chest when a lung is totally collapsed. Patients with pneumothorax generally note the rapid onset of pleuritic-type chest pain associated with some difficulty in breathing. There is hyperresonance to percussion on the side of lung collapse (see Chapter 3), and the trachea may deviate toward the opposite side of the chest.

Pleural Fluid

Fluid in the pleural cavity can accumulate as the result of excessive production, interference with the drainage mechanisms that normally keep the pleural space relatively dry, or a combination of both (Figure 1-13).

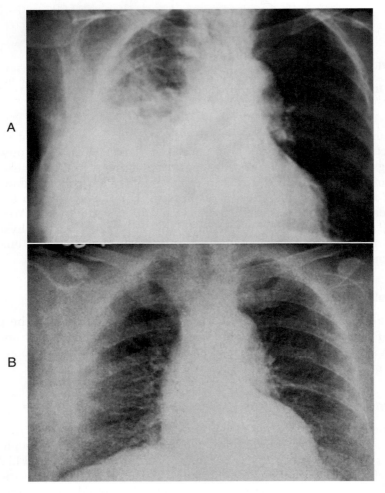

FIGURE 1-13. A, Radiograph demonstrating massive pleural effusion in right hemithorax in a cancer patient with pleural metastases. **B,** Film made 1 month after treatment. Patient's pleural effusion is diminished and shortness of breath relieved. (From Camishion RC, Gibbon JH, Nealon TF: *Surg Clin North Am* 42:1521, 1962.)

Inflammatory processes, alteration in venous or lymphatic flow, or changes in serum oncotic pressure can produce fluid accumulation between the pleural surfaces. Any substantial accumulation of fluid between these surfaces interferes with the transmission of breath sounds and vocal sounds; it also impairs resonance. When there is sufficient fluid accumulation to produce some compression of the underlying lung, the breath sound characteristics are altered (see Chapter 5). Breath sounds are absent over a large effusion.

Chapter Review and Critical Thinking Questions

1. *Why are aspirated fluids and inhaled foreign bodies more prone to enter the right lung?*

2. *What is the function of surfactant? What disease occurs when it is deficient?*

3. *During ordinary quiet breathing, why is muscle activity needed only for inspiration?*

4. *Describe a spirometer. What is its function?*

5. *What diseases commonly produce restricted pulmonary function?*

6. *What pulmonary function tests are used for estimating the degree of respiratory obstruction?*

7. *Which abnormalities tend to diminish the vital capacity?*

BIBLIOGRAPHY

Bates DV, Macklem PT, Christie RV: *Respiratory function in disease,* Philadelphia, 1971, WB Saunders.
Comroe JH: *The lung: clinical physiology and pulmonary function tests,* ed 2, Chicago, 1962, Mosby.
Comroe JH: *Physiology of respiration,* ed 2, Chicago, 1962, Mosby.
Divertie MB, Brass A, editors: *Respiratory system,* Summit, NJ, 1979, Ciba.
Guyton AC, Hall JE: *Textbook of medical physiology,* ed 10, Philadelphia, 2000, WB Saunders.
Hinshaw HC, Murray JF: *Diseases of the chest,* ed 4, Philadelphia, 1980, WB Saunders.
Prior JA, Silberstein JS: *Physical diagnosis,* ed 6, St Louis, 1981, Mosby.
West JB: *Respiratory physiology—the essentials,* ed 2, Baltimore, 1979, Williams & Wilkins.

Chapter 2

Sound, Hearing, and the Stethoscope

THE NATURE OF SOUND

Sounds consist of audible vibrations created by alternating regions of compression and rarefaction of air. To see what a sound wave looks like, one may mount a pen on one prong of a vibrating tuning fork and then run a piece of paper under the pen. The pen will inscribe an S-shaped wave called a *sine wave*. The peaks and valleys in the wave correspond to the alternating regions of compression and rarefaction that make up the sound wave (Figure 2-1).

Sound has three principal characteristics: frequency, intensity, and duration (Figure 2-2).

Frequency is a measure of the number of vibrations per unit time, in cycles per second or hertz (Hz). A large number of vibrations, as in a high-frequency wheeze, yield a sound that the examiner subjectively interprets as being high-pitched. A low-frequency wheeze, on the other hand, gives a sound that is heard as low-pitched.

Intensity is governed by four factors: (1) the amplitude of the vibrations, (2) the source producing the energy, (3) the distance the vibrations must travel, and (4) the medium through which they travel. These factors determine whether a sound is perceived as loud or faint. For example, breath sounds are much fainter than normal over an emphysematous lung because the damaged, hyperaerated tissue conducts sound poorly.

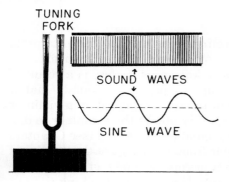

FIGURE 2-1. The vibrating tuning fork produces the sound wave shown *(top)*, which consists of alternating areas of compressed and rarefied air. The changing pressure in these areas corresponds to the sine wave below. (From Rushmer RF: *Cardiac diagnosis: a physiologic approach,* Philadelphia, 1955, WB Saunders.)

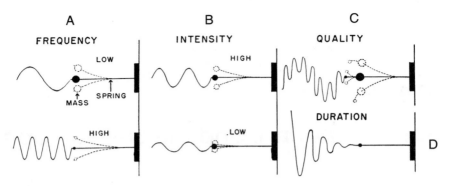

FIGURE 2-2. A, The frequency of vibration is determined by the relationship between mass and elasticity of the vibrating body; as shown in the example here, the larger mass *(upper drawing)* vibrates at a lower frequency. B, The amplitude of the vibration and the corresponding intensity of the sound depend on the amount of displacement of the vibrating body; a high-intensity sound is produced by a large displacement *(upper drawing)*. C, The quality or timbre of the sound is a result of the relative intensity of the component frequencies that make up the vibration. Shown here is a high-frequency sine wave (overtone) superimposed on a low-frequency sine wave (the fundamental). D, The duration of a vibration after the source of energy is cut off is dependent on the level of the energy and the rate at which it is dissipated. Note that each peak in the sine wave, going from left to right, is lower than the one before, indicating that the sound is diminishing progressively in amplitude. (From Rushmer RF: *Cardiac diagnosis: a physiologic approach,* Philadelphia, 1955, WB Saunders.)

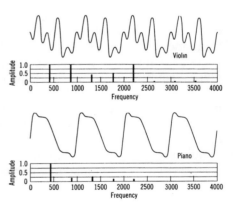

FIGURE 2-3. Wave form and sound spectrum for two stringed instruments—the violin and the piano. The fundamental frequency for both is 440 Hz (concert A). Four cycles of each wave are shown. The sound spectrum beneath each wave demonstrates the harmonic components of the wave. Note the presence of loud higher harmonics, especially the fifth, in the violin spectrum. (From Halliday D, Resnick R: *Physics,* New York, 1966, John Wiley & Sons.)

Duration of the vibrations determines whether the ear interprets them as short or long, for example, a short wheeze or a long wheeze.

A fourth characteristic, *quality,* also known as *timbre,* is a result of the component frequencies that make up any particular sound. Quality allows one to perceive the difference in the note A played on a violin or on a piano (Figure 2-3). In the chest, quality allows the examiner to distinguish between a vesicular and a bronchial breath sound (see Chapters 4 and 5). E to A egophony (see Chapter 5) occurs because the quality of the voice sound heard through the stethoscope depends on whether the sound is being transmitted through normal or consolidated lung tissue.

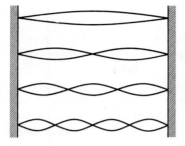

FIGURE 2-4. A vibrating string, fixed at both ends, showing the first four modes of vibration. The uppermost mode produces the fundamental tone; the lower three modes generate the overtones. (From Halliday D, Resnick R: *Physics*, New York, 1966, John Wiley & Sons.)

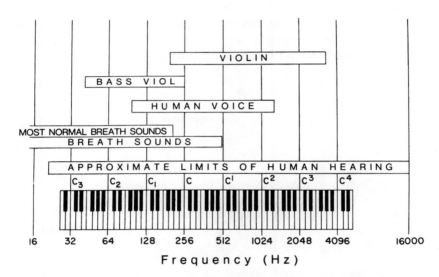

FIGURE 2-5. The frequency range of the piano keyboard and its relationship to the range of breath sounds. Note that most breath sounds fall into the region below 200 Hz. (Adapted from Butterworth JS, Chassin MR, McGrath R: *Cardiac auscultation including audio-visual principles*, New York, 1955, Grune & Stratton.)

Musical notes and breath sounds are made up of several frequency components. In a musical note, each of these components, which are simple multiples of one another, is called a *harmonic;* in most breath sounds, the relationship of the components is more complex, although a wheeze is quite analogous to a musical note. The pitch of a sound is determined by the component of lowest frequency, called the *fundamental*. The quality of a sound is determined by the higher-frequency components, called *overtones* in a musical sound (Figure 2-4).

In music, frequency or pitch is often expressed in terms of octaves above or below a given pitch, such as middle C. In the case of breath sounds, however, the number of cycles per second (Hz) is the preferred unit. The frequency range of the piano keyboard and its relationship to the range of breath sounds are shown in Figure 2-5.

HEARING

Most breath sounds fall into a frequency range to which the ear is relatively insensitive. Some of the basic physiology of hearing is presented to clarify this point.

The eardrum is mechanically coupled to the cochlear apparatus by the three tiny bones (malleus, incus, and stapes) of the middle ear, called the *ossicles* (Figure 2-6). The cochlea is essentially a selective sound frequency transducer, and a remarkably sensitive one. The eardrum need move only a distance equal to one tenth the diameter of a hydrogen molecule for sound to be heard.

The average young, healthy ear can detect sound vibrations with frequencies between approximately 16 and 16,000 Hz, although sensitivity varies greatly through this range. Maximum sensitivity is in the

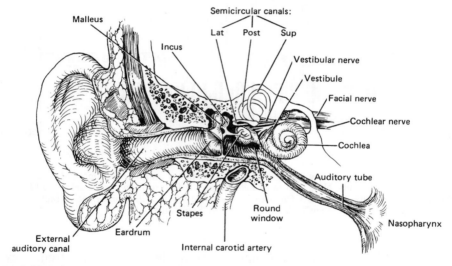

FIGURE 2-6. The human ear. Sound waves pass through the external auditory canal inward to the tympanic membrane, or eardrum. The middle ear is an air-filled cavity in the temporal bone that opens to the outside via the auditory tube and nasopharynx, the tube usually being closed. The three ossicles—the malleus, incus, and stapes—are located in the middle ear. The manubrium, or handle, of the malleus is attached to the back of the tympanic membrane; its head is attached to the wall of the middle ear, and its short process is attached to the incus, which in turn is joined to the head of the stapes (named for its resemblance to a stirrup). The faceplate of the stapes lies against the oval window; sound waves are transmitted from here into the cochlea. *Lat,* Lateral; *Post,* posterior; *Sup,* superior. To make the relationships clear, the cochlea has been turned slightly and the middle ear muscles have been omitted. (From Ganong WF: *Review of medical physiology,* ed 11, Los Altos, Calif, 1983, Lange Medical. Modified and redrawn from Brödel M: *Three unpublished drawings of the anatomy of the human ear.* Philadelphia, 1946, WB Saunders.)

region of 1000 to 2000 Hz. Below 1000 Hz, sensitivity falls off dramatically. For example, to be audible, a tone with a frequency of 100 Hz must have a sound pressure 100 times greater than a tone at 1000 Hz. Because most normal breath sounds are below 500 Hz, the ear is relatively insensitive to them and they are not heard as well as other types of sound (Figure 2-7).

An additional complexity of the frequency response characteristics of the ear is represented by the Fletcher-Munson phenomenon. At a high level of absolute intensity, sounds are more likely to be perceived by the ear as equally loud regardless of frequency composition. However, at a low level of absolute intensity, sounds seem to the ear to be higher pitched. The Fletcher-Munson phenomenon is not a factor when a stethoscope is being used. Yet it does affect the perception of recorded breath sounds played through a speaker; these sounds will seem unnaturally low-pitched and booming to the ear when compared with breath sounds heard through a stethoscope.

Because other sensory stimuli (noises, etc.) occurring during auscultation may dull auditory perception, the examiner should see to it that interference from such stimuli is reduced to a minimum. A good clinician listening for a faint sound through the stethoscope seeks as quiet a room as possible and also assumes a relaxed, comfortable position, sometimes with the eyes closed.

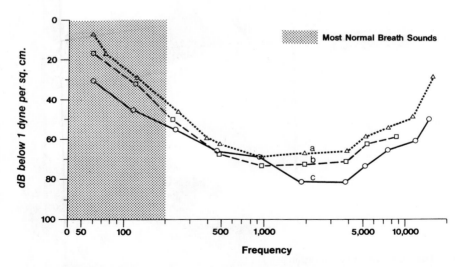

FIGURE 2-7. *A,* Threshold sensitivity (measured in decibels or dB) of the human ear for binaural hearing in a free field. *B,* Binaural hearing in a closed system analogous to the modern stethoscope. *C,* Monaural hearing in a closed system. Note that most breath sounds fall into the range in which the ear is least sensitive. (Modified from Weaver EG, Lawrence M: *Physiological acoustics,* Princeton, NJ, 1954, Princeton University Press.)

THE STETHOSCOPE

Since antiquity, physicians have listened to the sounds within the chest. The ancient Greeks recognized at least two characteristic sounds: (1) pleural friction rub, and (2) the splashing sound made by fluid within the chest cavity when the patient was shaken. Until the nineteenth century, the examiner detected these sounds by listening with the ear placed directly against the chest wall (Figure 2-8), despite the obvious drawbacks of patients' modesty and aversion to contact.

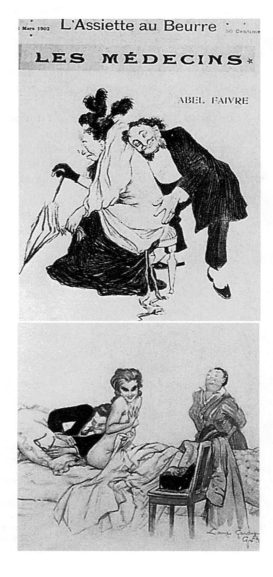

FIGURE 2-8. Direct auscultation of the chest, portrayed in two French caricatures. (From McKusick VA: *Cardiovascular sound in health and disease,* Baltimore, 1958, Williams & Wilkins.)

In 1816 a young French doctor, René Theophile Laennec, faced with examining the chest of a very obese woman, rolled a sheaf of paper into a cylinder; he placed one end on the patient's chest and put his ear to the other end (Figure 2-9). Laennec named his invention the stethoscope, from the Greek *stethos,* "breast," and *skopein,* "to view." He subsequently employed a wooden cylinder, and in 1819 he published a treatise on what he had learned with his instrument. Among his meticulous descriptions of sounds is the following: "When the patient coughed or spoke, and still more during respiration, there was heard a tinkling like that of a small bell which has just stopped ringing or of a gnat buzzing within a porcelain vase."

The modern stethoscope is often a combination of two types of chest pieces, tubing, a binaural headset, and eartips (Figure 2-10). These must function properly and fit well for best results. The open bell, or Ford chest piece, is similar to the old-fashioned trumpet-type hearing aid. It conducts sounds with practically no distortion. The bell is well suited for listening to low-pitched sounds. The closed diaphragm, or Bowles chest piece, has a larger diameter than the bell. The diaphragm is best suited for hearing high-pitched sounds, because it acts to attenuate low-frequency sounds and pass high-frequency sounds. But most stethoscopes

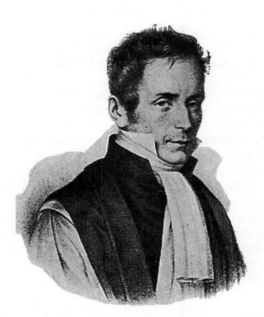

FIGURE 2-9. René Theophile Laennec (1781-1826) was a French physician who invented the stethoscope and gave the first accurate descriptions of normal and abnormal breath sounds, correlating them with pathologic autopsy findings. (From Garrison FH: *An introduction to the history of medicine,* ed 4, Philadelphia, 1929, WB Saunders.)

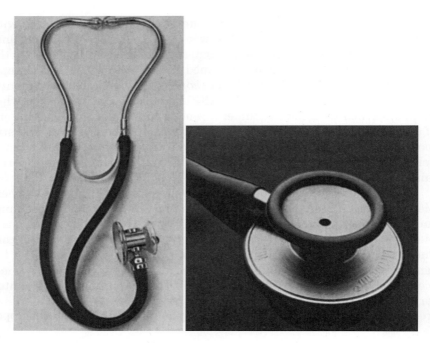

FIGURE 2-10. Two stethoscopes in common use today. (Courtesy Hewlett-Packard and 3M Company.)

tend to attenuate high-frequency sounds to some degree (Charbonneau and Sudraud, 1985).

Although not outwardly apparent, the bell chest piece is converted to a diaphragm chest piece when applied too tightly to the skin. The skin acts as the diaphragm.

The binaurals should be light and comfortable. The eartubes must be inclined anteriorly to conform to the direction of the normal ear canals. It is impossible to overemphasize the importance of a snug yet gentle fit at the ears; the best chest piece is completely unsatisfactory when joined to an uncomfortable headset and poorly fitting eartips.

Broken diaphragms should not be replaced by or improvised from any odd sheet material, such as x-ray film, which is not a good diaphragm substitute. A Bowles chest piece with either a makeshift or an absent diaphragm is a very poor instrument.

The examiner should periodically inspect the tubing for deterioration and holes by flexing it (Figure 2-11). Any damage to the tubing can render the stethoscope useless. But it is not good practice to replace the original flexible tubing with hospital tubing intended for other purposes. The manufacturer should be contacted for replacement tubing or other parts.

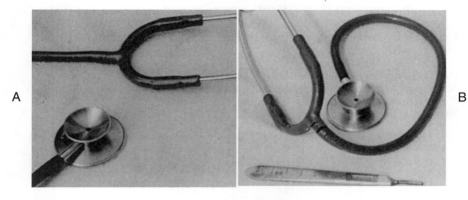

FIGURE 2-11. Detecting stethoscope damage. **A,** Stethoscope in unflexed position. **B,** Stethoscope in flexed position. Note holes in tubing. (From Orton D, Stryker R: *JAMA* 256:2817, 1986. Copyright 1986, American Medical Association.)

    In 1982, Dr. John Kindig and his associates published their acoustic tests of six popular, commercially available stethoscopes. Despite individual differences, they found no obviously superior model; in addition, a double-tube stethoscope held no advantage over a single-tube stethoscope. The listening ability of the examiner was far more important than the particular stethoscope being used.

Chapter Review and Critical Thinking Questions

1. *What are the principal characteristics of sound? What is the significance of each characteristic?*

2. *What determines the quality of a sound?*

3. *Which breath sound is analogous to a musical note?*

4. *Why are breath sounds more difficult to perceive than other types of sound?*

5. *To what type of sound is the bell chest piece on the stethoscope well suited? To what type of sound is the diaphragm chest piece best suited?*

BIBLIOGRAPHY

Charbonneau G, Sudraud M: Mesure de la réponse en fréquence de quelques stéthoscopes usuels: conséquences pour l'auscultation cardiaque et pulmonaire, *Bull Eur Physiopathol Respir* 21:49-54, 1985.
DeWeese D, Saunders WH: *Textbook of otolaryngology,* ed 5, St Louis, 1977, Mosby.

Kindig JR, Beeson TP, Campbell RW et al: Acoustical performance of the stetho-
scope: a comparative analysis, *Am Heart J* 104:269-275, 1982.
Littmann D: Stethoscopes and auscultation, *Am J Nurs* 72:1238-1241, 1972.
McKusick VA: *Cardiovascular sound in health and disease,* Baltimore, 1958,
Williams & Wilkins.
Orton D, Stryker R: Sick stethoscope syndrome, *JAMA* 256:2817, 1986.
Rappaport MB, Sprague B: The effects of tubing bore on stethoscope efficiency,
Am Heart J 42:605, 1951.
Reiser SJ: The medical influence of the stethoscope, *Sci Am* 240:148, 156, 1979.

Chapter 3

History and Physical Examination

A careful history and physical examination form the basis for all diagnosis of chest disease by medical and nursing personnel. Indeed, information so obtained may be the only readily available data, particularly on a new patient or a patient seen in the home. The results will often suggest further tests that should be performed.

HISTORY

Since most patients seek medical help because of symptoms, the clinical history is likely to furnish important clues to the presence of disease. Sometimes the history alone will facilitate a prompt diagnosis; more often, it will indicate an appropriate line of investigation. A careful history must be taken because events that seem of no significance to the patient may, in fact, be of crucial importance.

Chief Complaint

Why is the patient seeking medical attention? What seems to be the problem (e.g., cough, shortness of breath, abnormal chest radiograph on routine physical examination)? How long has the problem existed?

Family and Social History

The family and social history of patients with pulmonary disease is important for three reasons: (1) Some infections, notably tuberculosis, are transferred from person to person; therefore history of contact with an infected person, often an infected family member, may be elicited. (2) Allergic disorders, such as bronchial asthma, show an inherited predisposition. In addition, asthmatic attacks may be provoked by family and domestic conflict. (3) Chronic bronchitis patients may reside in a district with a high level of atmospheric pollution. However, air pollution worsens chronic bronchitis—it does not cause it.

Cigarette smoking is the most important cause of lung cancer, emphysema, and chronic bronchitis. All these conditions are quite rare in nonsmokers. The smoking history should contain the following details: (1) age when regular smoking started, (2) average number of cigarettes or cigars smoked per day or amount of pipe tobacco consumed per week, (3) age when smoking was given up (if applicable). Smoking history is often recorded in terms of pack-years. For example, a man who smoked two packs of cigarettes per day for 40 years would have an 80 pack-year smoking history.

Occupational History

Because both acute and chronic respiratory disease may result from certain types of dust inhaled at work, a complete occupational history must cover both present and previous employment. Industrial dusts may cause respiratory disease in coal miners, stone masons, arc welders, cotton handlers, potters, steel foundry workers, and farmworkers. Silica-bearing rock dust and asbestos, when inhaled, may not cause disease symptoms until years later. Thus occupational history must contain the degree and duration of exposure to dust and the time relationship of such exposure to the onset of symptoms. Equally important, although not invariably occupational, are elements in the patient's environment. For example, individuals in close contact with pigeons, parrots, parakeets, or canaries may develop allergic alveolitis or psittacosis. Persons with a family history of allergies may develop allergic rhinitis or bronchial asthma when exposed to such allergens as pollen, house dust, feathers, animal dander, or certain fungal spores. Persons who live and work in a particular part of the country may be exposed to certain pulmonary disease-causing agents. An example of such an illness is coccidioidomycosis, a systemic fungal disease, respiratory in origin, that spreads via the blood to subcutaneous tissues, bone, central nervous system, and skin and other organs. Exposure to histoplasmosis, another systemic fungal disease, is common in some parts of the eastern and midwestern United States.

History of Previous Illness

In a patient with respiratory illness, valuable information may lie in the medical history, especially with regard to the diseases and circumstances discussed in the following sections.

Tuberculosis
Pulmonary tuberculosis in childhood may cause bronchiectasis in later life; if inadequately treated, tuberculosis may later relapse. Advanced tuberculosis of both lungs can produce severe fibrosis, leading to respiratory failure and heart failure. Bronchiectasis at the site of an inactive tu-

berculous lesion may be associated with the coughing up of blood. Patients should be asked about prior vaccination with bacille Calmette-Guérin (BCG); when successful, this vaccination gives considerable protection against tuberculosis.

Pneumonia

A few chronic pulmonary disorders, such as bronchiectasis, may begin after an episode of pneumonia, described by some patients as "pleurisy." Recurrent pneumonia, occurring in the same side of the chest, suggests bronchiectasis or lung cancer. Pneumonia is also a common problem of children with cystic fibrosis.

Chest Injuries and Operations

The circumstances of some chest injuries and operations may suggest that they are related to the present illness. For example, accidental or surgical trauma may produce a chest wall deformity. A metal foreign body, such as a bullet or shrapnel fragment, lodged in the lung may cause recurrent coughing up of blood or development of a pulmonary abscess. A traumatic hemothorax, particularly if complicated by infection, may cause gross thickening of the pleura.

PAIN

A history of chest pain frequently causes a patient to seek medical advice. The various forms of thoracic pain may be classified as follows:

Pulmonary Pain—Primary and Referred

The lung tissue and the visceral pleura covering it are insensitive to pain. Even large tumors involving these regions may cause little or no discomfort. However, pain does occur when a pathologic process affects the parietal pleura (covering the interior of the chest wall), major airways, chest wall, diaphragm, or mediastinal structures.

Like other forms of pain, thoracic pain may be referred to an area of skin supplied by similar nerve roots arising from the spinal cord. Thus pain originating within the chest may cause anterior upper abdominal pain where the intercostal nerves innervate the abdominal wall. Another example is the referral of pain arising in the diaphragmatic pleura to the base of the neck and shoulder; these regions are supplied by the third, fourth, and fifth cervical nerve roots, which also make up the phrenic nerve.

Esophageal disease can cause referred thoracic pain. Esophageal spasm, achalasia, hiatus hernia, esophagitis, or carcinoma of the esophagus may be confused with cardiac and lung pathology; they all produce a similar type of pain.

Pleural Pain

Acute inflammation of the parietal pleura and viral pleuritis may cause intense pain (pleurodynia). Pneumonia, pulmonary embolism, tuberculosis, and malignant disease all can cause pleuritic pain, which is localized rather than diffuse. The relationship of such pain to motions of the thorax prompts patients to describe it as a severe "catch" in the side of the chest, preventing them from breathing freely; they quickly learn that when they limit chest expansion, the pain is reduced. Motion of the trunk—bending, stooping, turning in bed—aggravates the pain; coughing and sneezing can provoke exquisite distress. Diagnostic possibilities are suggested by details of the pain history. Severe pleural pain several days after major surgery may signal a pulmonary embolus. However, the same pain associated with acute respiratory infection, fever, cough, and expectoration can indicate acute pneumonia. In a prolonged illness that is characterized by weight loss, depletion of energy, and persistent cough, pleural pain may indicate tuberculosis or chest malignancy. Pleural pain may not be distinguishable from pulmonary pain.

Pain of Intercostal Neuritis

Intercostal neuritis, especially when caused by herpes zoster (shingles), may cause pain that is similar to that of pleuritis. However, neuritic pain is more likely to be superficial in character and related to coughing, sneezing, or straining but not to other movements; these characteristics are especially prominent when the neural pain is caused by a tumor of the spinal cord. The pain of intercostal neuritis is often described as an electric shock sensation, unrelated to the movements of respiration, and is sometimes associated with hypersensitive or anesthetic areas of skin on the chest wall.

Muscular Pain

Sometimes even a skilled examiner can temporarily mistake the symptoms of acute inflammation of the muscles of the chest wall, accepting them as evidence of disease within the chest. Local tenderness frequently provides a clue to the correct diagnosis.

Costochondral Pain

In the condition that produces costochondral pain, called *Tietze's syndrome,* there is tenderness on pressure and palpable enlargement of the cartilages that lie between the ribs and the sternum. Afflicted patients may fear that they have serious cardiac or pulmonary disease. The second, third, and fourth cartilages are most often affected, but any part of the large cartilaginous shield along the lower border of the thoracic cage may be involved. The pain is dull, frequently described as gnawing or aching; it bears little relationship to movement and is most noticeable when the patient is lying in bed at night. Although mild, the pain may persist for many months or years.

Cardiac, Pericardial, and Aortic Pain and Pain of Pulmonary Embolus

Cardiac pain is in many cases so characteristic that it can be diagnosed on the basis of history alone. The patient feels it as a "crushing pain," lying beneath the sternum and to the left, radiating into the shoulders, arms, or neck. Cardiac pain caused by exertion or anxiety, relieved by rest or nitroglycerin, is typical of angina pectoris. The pain of an acutely occluded coronary artery may be confused with conditions affecting the abdomen and the thorax; it is retrosternal and is associated with shock, enzyme elevations, and electrocardiographic changes. Pericardial pain, like cardiac pain, is retrosternal, extending to the left side, and, like angina, may be related to exertion. However, it is also affected by respiration and therefore is similar to pleural pain. Typically, the patient's pain is relieved by sitting up and leaning forward.

Aortic pain caused by an aneurysm, especially a dissecting one, is described by the patient as a deep, boring, agonizing, tearing pain; it may be compared with the pain of a severe toothache. The location is retrosternal or, sometimes, interscapular.

Pulmonary embolus may sometimes produce pain along with shortness of breath, hemoptysis (rarely), and cough.

COUGH

Cough is a cardinal sign of pulmonary disease (Figure 3-1). Secretions of the bronchial mucosa are constantly produced and flow in an orderly manner from smaller to larger airways; they are propelled by tiny, fingerlike structures called *cilia*. Finally, they ascend the trachea, mix with saliva, and are swallowed. In normal persons, all this is accomplished without cough. Therefore, any cough suggests an abnormality—possibly trivial, perhaps critical.

There are basically two types of cough: productive and nonproductive. A productive cough clears the airways of the viscous secretions that accumulate in many pulmonary disorders. Nonproductive cough is an irritative phenomenon and serves no useful purpose; the stimulus for it may be mechanical or chemical, including inflammatory reactions.

A loose cough accompanied by a low-pitched, rattling sound is often associated with heavy smoking habits, history of bronchitis, copious daily sputum volume, and relatively poor performance in forced expiratory

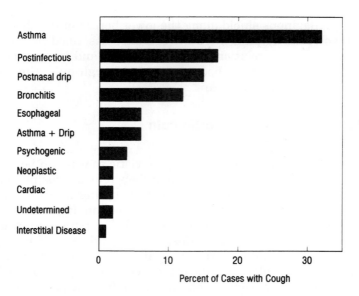

FIGURE 3-1. Causes of chronic cough in two series of patients (158 patients total). Percentage does not equal 100 because of rounding of numbers. (From Irwin RS, Corrao WM, Pratter MR: *Am Rev Resp Dis* 123:413-417, 1981; Poe RH, Israel RH, Utell MJ et al: *Am Rev Resp Dis* 126:160-162, 1982. Data tabulated in Murray JF: Diagnostic evaluation: history and physical examination. In Murray JF, Nadel JA, editors: *Textbook of respiratory medicine,* Philadelphia, 1988, WB Saunders.)

tests. The source of the rattling sound is presumably the passage of gas through airways that are lightly occluded.

The type of sputum produced is suggestive of the pathologic process. Foul-smelling sputum is often found in anaerobic bacterial infection—lung abscess, for example. Abundant, frothy, salivalike sputum is a rare but characteristic symptom of bronchioloalveolar carcinoma. Voluminous, pink, frothy sputum is seen in patients with pulmonary edema. Pneumococcal pneumonia is often associated with rust-colored sputum. Copious purulent sputum, brought up on change of posture, may indicate bronchiectasis.

At times, severe episodes of coughing can progress to muscular exhaustion and unconsciousness, called *cough syncope.* This condition is usually found in strong, middle-aged men who smoke excessively. Chronic bronchitis and asthma also are frequently present. Although the cause is unknown, hyperventilation with excessive loss of carbon dioxide from the blood is suspected.

HEMOPTYSIS

Hemoptysis, the coughing up of blood, is a frightening experience that usually causes a patient to seek medical advice without delay. Small

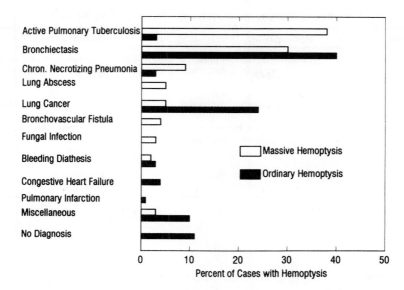

FIGURE 3-2. Comparison of causes of "ordinary" and "massive" hemoptysis from two series of 129 and 123 patients, respectively. (From Gong H, Salvatierra C: *Am Rev Resp Dis* 124:221-225, 1981; Conlan AA, Hurwitz SS, Kriege L et al: *J Thorac Cardiovasc Surg* 85:120-124, 1983. Data tabulated in Murray JF: Diagnostic evaluation: history and physical examination. In Murray JF, Nadel JA, editors: *Textbook of respiratory medicine,* Philadelphia, 1988, WB Saunders.)

streaks of blood may appear in the sputum of patients with acute respiratory tract infections, while patients with pneumonia may cough up grossly bloody sputum. Some patients who expectorate bloody sputum are seriously ill; they may have bronchiectasis, tuberculosis, mitral stenosis, or bronchogenic carcinoma. Most commonly, they have bronchitis (Figure 3-2).

In many cases, the patient is unaware of the origin of the blood and will commonly state that it just "welled up" in his or her throat. Although the blood may occasionally come from a source in the nasopharynx, most commonly it originates either from the gastrointestinal tract (hematemesis) or from the lung.

Bleeding from esophageal varices may be confused with hemoptysis. Usually, however, blood is vomited during variceal bleeding, and the patient subsequently notes black stools. Other features distinguishing hemoptysis from hematemesis are noted in Table 3-1.

DYSPNEA

Dyspnea, or difficult breathing, is most often described by patients as shortness of breath. Because breathing is such a primitive, urgent human

TABLE 3-1. Differential Diagnosis of Hemoptysis and Hematemesis

Feature	Hemoptysis	Hematemesis
Prodrome	Tingling in throat, desire to cough	Nausea, stomach distress
Onset	Blood is coughed up; retching may accompany	Blood is vomited; coughing may accompany
Appearance	Some portions frothy	Never frothy
Color	Portions may be bright red	Uniformly dark red
pH reaction	Alkaline	Acid
Content	Leukocytes, microorganisms, hemosiderin-laden macrophages	Food particles
Past history	Lung disease	Alcoholism, peptic ulcer, liver disease
Anemia	Occasionally present	Common
Stools (at onset)	Guaiac negative	Guaiac positive

From Hinshaw HC, Murray JF: *Diseases of the chest*, ed 4, Philadelphia, 1980, WB Saunders.

need, dyspnea is more profoundly disturbing to the patient than almost any other symptom.

Circumstances associated with the dyspnea should be carefully noted by the examiner. Is the dyspnea associated with exertion? Does it occur after the patient walks half a block or climbs one flight of stairs? Dyspnea accompanied by wheezing may result from exercise-induced asthma. Although paroxysmal nocturnal dyspnea is a sign of left ventricular failure, it may sometimes be confused with bronchial asthma. Sudden, unprovoked dyspnea may result from spontaneous pneumothorax, pulmonary embolism, or myocardial infarction. Many patients with advanced lung disease also complain of paroxysmal nocturnal dyspnea and orthopnea.

In addition, the emotional state of the patient must be taken into account; shortness of breath, not related to exertion and not caused by organic disease but associated with anxiety states, is a common complaint. The patient will say that the air "doesn't go deep enough," that he or she cannot get enough air, and that the sense of air hunger is difficult to relieve, even with deep, sighing breaths. During the interview, the irregular breathing habits and occasional deep sighs will be apparent to the examiner. Although the diagnosis is usually obvious, a thorough examination, including pulmonary function tests, should be performed.

Some very emotional patients with psychogenic air hunger will hyperventilate, reducing dissolved arterial carbon dioxide below normal. This condition is encountered frequently. The increasingly forceful, rapid breathing is followed by numbness of the extremities, tingling sensations around the mouth, and mild clouding of consciousness, but rarely complete syncope. The diagnosis is made by asking the patient to breathe deeply and rapidly for 1 to 2 minutes and then to compare the symptoms produced with those that occur during spontaneous attacks.

HOARSENESS AND WHEEZE

Hoarseness is usually the result of an abnormality of the larynx and vocal cords. Occasionally, however, hoarseness may be the result of a lung tumor or aortic aneurysm that damages the recurrent laryngeal nerve, resulting in left vocal cord paralysis.

When a patient complains of wheeze, he or she may have various conditions in mind. Some persons use "wheeze" to describe noisy and labored breathing; others apply it to rattling secretions in the upper airways. However, wheeze usually denotes the musical sounds that are described more fully in Chapter 5. Many patients become so accustomed to wheezing that they cease to be cognizant of it unless it is called to their attention. The patient should be asked when the wheeze is present and whether it is made worse by exertion, inhalation of dust, or a respiratory infection.

Some patients with stridor, which is discussed fully in Chapter 5, may describe it as a wheeze. Care must be taken to differentiate between these two sounds. Stridor, a high-pitched musical or "crowing" sound, usually results from obstruction of a major airway; it demands urgent investigation and treatment.

PHYSICAL EXAMINATION

Every examiner should develop a routine, a specific sequence in which the procedures of physical examination—inspection, palpation, percussion, and auscultation—are performed. The learning of a routine ensures that no aspect of the examination is forgotten. Usually, the blood pressure is measured first, after which the heart rate is determined while a thermometer is in the patient's mouth to register body temperature. The remainder of the examination may then proceed.

Inspection

To begin, the patient should be unclothed to the waist. The room should be well lighted. Above all, both the patient and the examiner should be in comfortable positions; if either is uncomfortable, the examination will be hurried and, as a consequence, less thorough.

The examiner should first note whether the patient is breathless when talking or whether he or she is able to articulate long sentences without stopping to breathe. Hoarseness and stridor should be obvious at this time. Normal breathing is quiet except for occasional sighs; audible wheezing indicates severe bronchospasm. The gurgling of secretions suggests mucous retention, and endotracheal suction may be necessary.

Observation of the sputum is mandatory. It should be inspected for color, odor, and the presence of mucous plugs. If a cup is present at the bedside, the amount produced over 24 hours should be noted; any increase may suggest a worsening of the patient's condition.

If the patient is coughing, the nature of the cough should be noted. A weak cough may be the result of weakness or paralysis of respiratory muscles, anesthesia, or use of sedatives or narcotics. Patients with a weak cough are prone to mucous retention, atelectasis, and abnormal blood gas levels because of their inability to cough up secretions. A dry, hacking cough suggests airway irritation.

Skin Color

The skin, mucous membranes, conjunctiva, soft palate, lips, and tongue should be observed to detect cyanosis and pallor. Cyanosis is a bluish or grayish tinge to the skin and fingernails that is caused by diminished oxygen content of the blood; when especially marked, cyanosis may indicate impending cardiorespiratory collapse. Pallor, a paleness of the skin, may indicate anemia or chronic illness; however, some healthy people are normally quite pale. In advanced pulmonary disease, patients may develop a reddish-blue tint to the skin, the result of increased total hemoglobin and increased unoxygenated hemoglobin.

Neck Vein Distention

In chronic obstructive pulmonary disease, the neck veins distend on expiration and collapse on inspiration, especially in a very breathless patient. Expiratory distention is the result of positive pressure in the chest from increased work of breathing; inspiratory collapse occurs as negative pressure within the thorax facilitates the return of venous blood to the heart. If the patient has right ventricular heart failure and pulmonary disease, the inspiratory collapse may not occur.

Extremities

The fingers and fingernails should be examined for evidence of clubbing and tobacco stains. Clubbing, an abnormality of the nails and distal phalanges, causes bulbous changes of the fingertips and toes (Figure 3-3). Although clubbing may be a normal familial trait, it is often seen in patients with congenital heart disease, subacute bacterial endocarditis, bronchiectasis, cystic fibrosis, lung abscess, pulmonary fibrosis, lung cancer, liver cirrhosis, chronic ulcerative colitis, and regional enteritis.

Early clubbing can be detected by noting whether or not the normal slight angle is present between the nail and the finger (Figure 3-4). In early clubbing, this angle is lost, and the base of the nail bed will feel soft and spongy. As the condition progresses, the nail feels as though it is floating in a bed of soft vascular tissue. In advanced clubbing, the nail takes on a so-called watch glass deformity, and the fingertips become wider and rounder; the overlying skin stretches, loses normal wrinkles, and has a polished, glistening appearance.

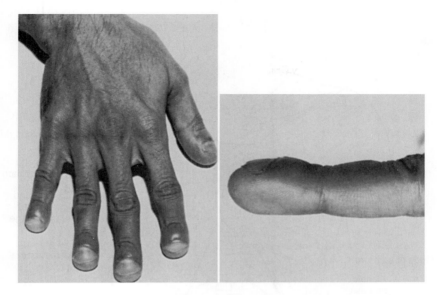

FIGURE 3-3. Top view of the right hand and side view of the index finger of a patient with advanced clubbing resulting from interstitial lung disease. (From Hinshaw HC, Murray JF: *Diseases of the chest,* ed 4, Philadelphia, 1980, WB Saunders.)

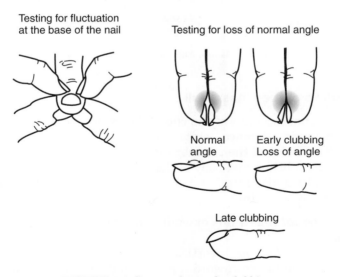

FIGURE 3-4. Signs and tests for clubbing.

Hypertrophic pulmonary osteoarthropathy is characterized pathologically by bilateral subperiosteal bone formation along long and tubular bones. Deformity of the digits is associated with enlarged ankles, wrists, interphalangeal joints of the fingers and toes, and distal ends of the long bones in the arms and legs. This condition is most common in lung cancer.

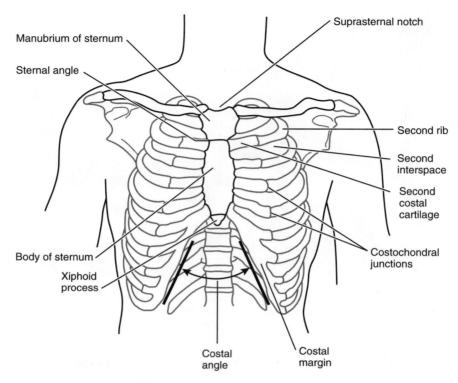

FIGURE 3-5. Anatomy of the chest wall.

Examination of the Chest Wall

To describe abnormalities of the chest, the examiner should be aware of certain anatomic reference points (Figure 3-5). The suprasternal notch marks the top point of the manubrium. The sternal angle is the point at which the manubrium and body of the sternum join; the anterior portion of the second rib also attaches here. Figure 3-6 shows these additional anatomic reference points:

- *Midsternal line:* a line extending downward from the sternal notch
- *Midclavicular line:* a vertical line parallel to the midsternal line and extending downward from the midpoint of each clavicle
- *Anterior axillary line:* a line extending downward from the anterior axillary fold
- *Posterior axillary line:* a line parallel to the anterior axillary line beginning at the posterior axillary fold
- *Midaxillary line:* a vertical line starting at a point midway between the anterior and posterior axillary lines

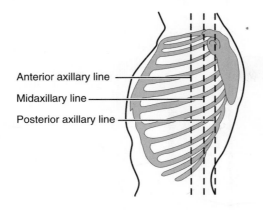

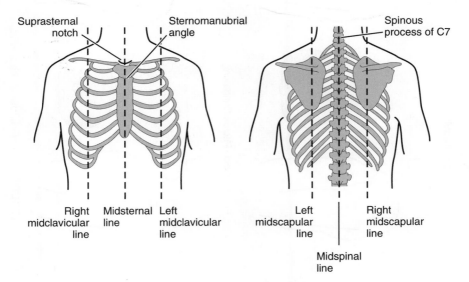

FIGURE 3-6. Thoracic cage landmarks.

- *Midspinal line:* a vertical line in the center of the back running along the spinal processes
- *Midscapular lines:* vertical lines on the back, parallel to the midspinal line, extending through the apices of the scapulae
- *Infrascapular area:* area of the posterior thorax lying below the scapulae
- *Interscapular area:* area of the posterior thorax lying between the scapulae

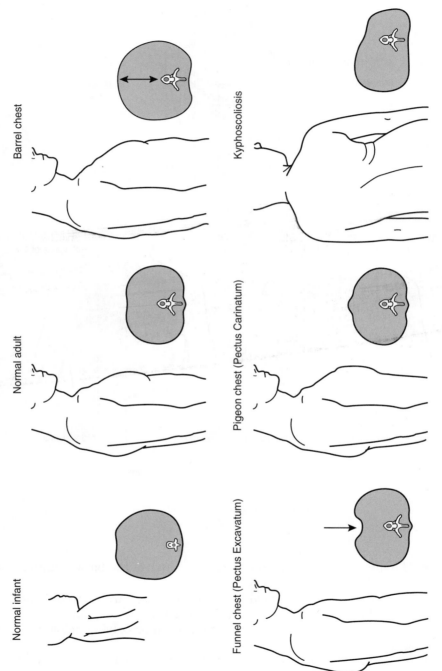

FIGURE 3-7. Deformities of the thorax.

Using these landmarks, the examiner should record the site of an identifying mark, percussion abnormality, auscultatory sound, or other change as, for example, "5 cm to the right of the midsternal line at the level of the fourth rib."

Certain abnormalities in the shape of the chest should be noted (Figure 3-7):

1. Increase in anteroposterior diameter relative to lateral diameter. This ratio varies in normal persons from about 5:7 to 1:2. However, in patients with chronic obstructive pulmonary disease, primarily emphysema, the anteroposterior dimension of the chest may increase to such an extent that the ratio of the two dimensions approximates 1:1, a condition referred to as *barrel chest*. Care should be taken to distinguish barrel chest from kyphosis, an abnormally increased curvature of the spine that also increases the anteroposterior diameter.

2. Pectus carinatum, or "pigeon breast," is commonly the result of chronic respiratory disease in childhood. It is characterized by a localized prominence of the sternum and adjacent rib cartilages, often associated with indrawn ribs forming symmetric horizontal grooves (Harrison's sulci) above the usually everted rib margins.

3. Pectus excavatum, or "funnel chest," is a congenital abnormality, a localized depression of the lower end of the sternum, or, uncommonly, depression of the entire sternum and the attached rib cartilages. Pectus excavatum generally is asymptomatic; however, when severe, the ventilatory capacity of the lungs may be diminished, accompanied by heart murmurs and other disturbances in cardiac function.

4. Kyphosis, an increase in the normal curvature of the thoracic spine, causes the patient to appear hunched over or hunchbacked. Although now frequently associated with the osteoporosis of the aging process, kyphosis is also seen in spinal tuberculosis (Pott's disease); it results from the inflammation-induced vertebral deformity. Kyphosis appears in persons with rheumatoid arthritis, Paget's disease, acromegaly, or many years of poor posture.

   Kyphosis, although usually an increased curvature of the spine, may also appear in the form of an *angular kyphosis*—a protruding hump in the back resulting from the collapse of one or more vertebral bodies. The hump, called a *gibbus,* may accompany tuberculosis of the spine or any other condition producing compression fractures of the vertebrae.

5. Scoliosis is a lateral curvature of the thoracic spine, accompanied by vertebral rotation. The disc spaces become narrower on the concave side of the curve and wider on the convex side. The vertebral bodies become wedged and are thicker on the convex side.

In most cases of scoliosis, called *idiopathic scoliosis,* the cause is unknown, although about 90% of these are genetic and hereditary. Some cases are caused by congenital vertebral deformity, poliomyelitis, neurofibromatosis, or juvenile rheumatoid arthritis. Idiopathic scoliosis occurs approximately seven times more often in girls than in boys. It is classified as infantile, juvenile, and adult types, according to well-defined peak periods of onset.

Infantile idiopathic scoliosis begins between birth and 3 years of age. It is more common in males, and the majority of cases resolve spontaneously, even if not treated.

Juvenile idiopathic scoliosis occurs between the ages of 4 and 10. It is more evenly distributed between the sexes, most cases being recognized when the patient is about 6 years old.

Adolescent idiopathic scoliosis consists of those cases diagnosed between age 10 and skeletal maturity. Seventy percent of affected children are girls. In general, all cases of scoliosis tend to progress most rapidly during the years of adolescent growth.

In mild cases of scoliosis, there is a single lateral curve, usually toward the right. In more severe cases, there is a thoracic curve and a compensatory lumbar curve, causing an S-shaped or backward S-shaped deformity of the spine. Severe scoliosis is readily apparent in the standing patient. Milder cases can be identified by the elevated shoulder and humping of ribs on one side of the back when the patient bends forward.

Scoliosis is a significant finding in the patient with chest disease because of the respiratory impairment associated with severe spinal deformity. The curvature and rotation of the spine cause advancing respiratory restriction later in life; these patients may die of severe pneumonia superimposed on the preexisting respiratory impairment.

In all advanced cases of scoliosis, breath sounds are diminished on the side of the chest in which the ribs are crowded together, reflecting the poor alveolar ventilation and air flow.

6. Kyphoscoliosis is a combination of backward and lateral curvature of the spine. Of all spinal deformities, this one causes the most serious physical impairment of the heart and lungs. Many patients have severe cardiac and respiratory failure by middle age.

In addition to these abnormalities in the shape of the chest, certain chest wall lesions should also be mentioned:

1. Skin abnormalities—eruptions, nodules, purple spots or bruises, scars of surgery or trauma.
2. Subcutaneous changes—particularly swellings. Subcutaneous emphysema, the presence of air in the subcutaneous tissues,

may result in diffuse swelling of the chest wall, the neck, and, uncommonly, the face. The air-filled tissues have a characteristic crackling sensation when palpated. Subcutaneous emphysema of the chest usually occurs when air from a tension pneumothorax escapes along the track of a needle or catheter used to decompress the pleural space. When alveoli rupture, air can also escape into the mediastinum, causing mediastinal emphysema.

3. Other chest wall abnormalities—spider telangiectases (dilation of small vessels) in liver disease; enlarged blood vessels (veins in superior vena cava syndrome, arteries in coarctation of the aorta); localized prominences and bone deformities.

Tracheal position should be midline; this is discussed more fully in the section on palpation.

Observation of Respiratory Motions

A normal adult takes about 14 breaths per minute. While the subject is breathing quietly, the examiner should observe the chest wall for symmetric bilateral expansion; this observation is best made with the subject lying supine and the examiner watching from the foot of the bed. If there is asymmetry, decreased size, or restricted expansion of one side of the thorax, disease may be present, for example, thickened fibrotic pleura, pleural inflammation, or trauma such as a fractured rib.

If the patient is breathing abnormally, the examiner should record the exact abnormality. *Bradypnea,* an abnormal slowing of respiration, may result from oxygen toxicity, primary hypoventilation, opiates, or brain tumor. *Apnea* is a temporary cessation of respiration. *Tachypnea,* an increased respiratory rate, may be seen in fever, pneumonia, or metabolic alkalosis; it is also seen in anxiety states and after exercise. *Hyperpnea,* an increase in the depth of respiration, is sometimes called *air hunger* and is frequently associated with metabolic acidosis. *Periodic respiration,* which is alternating hyperpnea and apnea, may be present in relatively serious disease states, although it is occasionally observed as a nonpathologic occurrence in child and in the normal sleeping adult.

One variant of periodic respiration, Cheyne-Stokes breathing, was originally described in a case report by John Cheyne himself, as follows: "His breathing was irregular; it would entirely cease for a quarter of a minute, then it would become perceptible, though very low, then by degrees it became heaving and quick, and then it would gradually cease again. This revolution in the state of his breathing occupied about a minute, during which there were about 30 acts of respiration." This form of breathing takes place when the brain's respiratory center in the medulla and the regulating corticobulbar tracts lose their usual fine sensitivity to fluctuations in carbon dioxide tension or nervous stimuli; it is most common in cerebral disorders such as cerebrovascular accidents; it is also seen in brain tumor, heart disease, chronic kidney disease, meningitis, and pneumonia.

A striking form of abnormal breathing, Biot's respiration, may be seen in meningitis and medullary lesions. Camille Biot first described it as follows: "This irregularity of the respiratory movements is not periodic, sometimes slow, sometimes rapid, sometimes superficial, sometimes deep, but without any constant relation of succession between the two types, with pauses following irregular intervals, preceded and often followed by a sigh more or less prolonged."

Another abnormal breathing pattern is *sighing respiration*. Sighing respiration is characterized by deep inspiration interrupting the normal respiratory rhythm, often accompanied by an audible sigh. This form of breathing is almost always a sign of emotional tension and is rarely associated with organic disease. Spirograms of some of the breathing patterns described here are presented in Figure 3-8.

Besides respiratory rhythm, pulmonary disease may affect the mode of breathing. In normal persons, as is mentioned in Chapter 1, inspiration is mediated by contraction of the external intercostal muscles and the diaphragm, whereas expiration is passive, dependent on the elastic recoil of the lungs. Women tend to use the intercostal muscles, whereas men

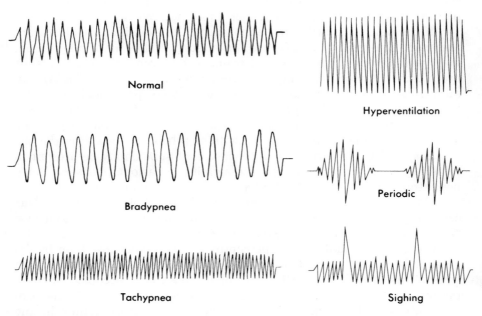

Normal

Hyperventilation

Bradypnea

Periodic

Tachypnea

Sighing

FIGURE 3-8. Spirograms of normal, slow, and rapid respiration *(left),* and altered respiration *(right).* (From Prior JA: Thorax and lungs. In Prior JA, Silberstein JS, Stang JM, editors: *Physical diagnosis,* ed 6, St Louis, 1981, Mosby.)

and infants of both sexes use the diaphragm. These departures from the norm should be recorded:

1. If the mode of breathing is exclusively thoracic and confined to the intercostal muscles, the examiner should suspect that diaphragmatic movement is inhibited by the following: (a) peritoneal irritation; (b) severe abdominal distention from ascites, gaseous distention of the bowel, a large ovarian cyst, or pregnancy; or (c) diaphragmatic paralysis.
2. If the mode of breathing is exclusively abdominal, lack of chest expansion may be to the result of ankylosing spondylitis, intercostal paralysis, or pleural pain.

As mentioned in Chapter 1, patients use the accessory muscles of respiration—sternocleidomastoids, scaleni, and trapezii—when pulmonary function is compromised and adequate ventilation is not possible. These muscles lift the ribs out and up with every breath and are used in such conditions as advanced emphysema, severe bronchial asthma, and obstruction of the larynx and trachea. Moreover, such breathing is often accompanied by retraction of the suprasternal and supraclavicular fossae, the intercostal spaces, and the epigastrium with each inspiration.

Even more retraction of the chest wall is present in patients who have sustained a series of double fractures of the ribs or sternum (flail chest). The region of chest wall between the fractures becomes mobile and is sucked in with each inspiration. This *paradoxical movement* gravely hampers pulmonary ventilation and thus may be accompanied by severe respiratory distress and hypoxia. In addition to the abnormal inspiratory movements already described, abnormal expiratory movements may result from strong contractions of the abdominal muscles and latissimus dorsi, particularly if elastic recoil of the lungs is not sufficient to fully expel air from the alveoli. These abnormal expiratory movements are seen in some types of emphysema or in cases in which expiratory airway obstruction is present—bronchial asthma and some forms of chronic bronchitis, for example. Patients so afflicted sit upright, holding the bed table or back of a chair, fixing the shoulder girdle so that the latissimus dorsi can be used to approximate the ribs and augment the respiratory effort. In addition, these patients purse their lips during expiration to keep the intrabronchial pressure above that in the adjacent alveoli, preventing collapse of the bronchial walls.

PALPATION

A considerable amount of information pertinent to the thorax and lungs can be gathered by palpation; the knowledge gained by history and inspection may be supplemented.

One of the most important functions of palpation is the careful search for lymph nodes. The examiner should palpate the cervical nodal

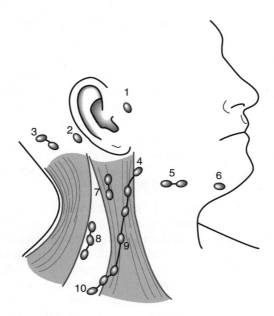

FIGURE 3-9. Lymph node regions of the neck. *1,* Preauricular—in front of the ear; *2,* posterior auricular—superficial to the mastoid process; *3,* occipital—at the base of the skull posteriorly; *4,* tonsillar—at the angle of the mandible; *5,* submaxillary—halfway between the angle and the tip of the mandible; *6,* submental—in the midline behind the tip of the mandible; *7,* superficial cervical—superficial to the sternomastoid; *8,* posterior cervical chain—along the anterior edge of the trapezius; *9,* deep cervical chain—deeper than the sternomastoid and often inaccessible to examination. To find these lymph nodes, the examiner hooks the thumb and fingers around either side of the sternomastoid muscle; *10,* supraclavicular—deep in the angle formed by the clavicle and sternomastoid.

chains and the supraclavicular regions on both sides, rolling the skin over underlying structures, first lightly, then more heavily, to locate any nodes, superficial or deep. Even the smallest node may prove to be of paramount significance; biopsy of such a node may be the only practical means of making a diagnosis of lung cancer (Figure 3-9).

The axillary nodes should be examined with great care. The examiner should bear the weight of the patient's relaxed arm; one hand is then placed at the elbow, the other reaches high into the axillary space. The group of nodes usually found in this region should be rolled under the fingers.

The trachea is palpated to detect any deviation from its normal position in the middle of the neck. If one lung is atelectatic, the trachea will be displaced to the side of the abnormality, particularly on inspiration (Figure 3-10). Fixed lateral displacement of the trachea may be the result of aortic aneurysm, mediastinal tumor, neck tumor, unilaterally enlarged paratracheal lymph nodes, or unilateral thyroid enlargement. The tra-

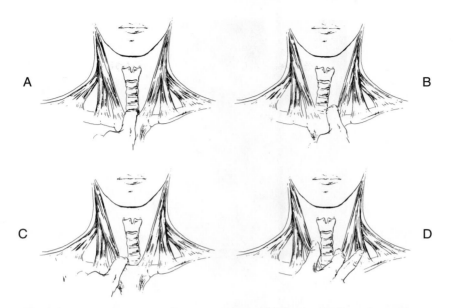

FIGURE 3-10. Determining the position of the trachea. **A,** With the patient's neck flexed and chin in the midline position, check for anterior displacement of the trachea (shallow suprasternal notch) by inserting fingertip directly in the middle of the suprasternal notch. Inability to place a fingertip into this notch indicates anterior displacement. **B** and **C,** Check for lateral displacement of the trachea by firmly inserting the index finger in the suprasternal notch, first on the left side and then on the right. The spaces should feel symmetric. **D,** Some clinicians prefer to check for tracheal deviation by palpating with the thumb and forefinger.

chea will deviate on expiration from the affected hemithorax in tension pneumothorax, large hemothorax, or pleural effusion. Anterior displacement of the trachea, indicated by a suprasternal notch into which a fingertip cannot be inserted, is seen in tumor behind the trachea, some cases of goiter, and dilated esophagus in achalasia. Palpable voice-generated vibrations transmitted to the chest wall are called *tactile fremitus* or *vocal fremitus*. To elicit this sign, the examiner asks the patient to count "one, two, three" or say "ninety-nine." The palpating hand is placed, palm against the chest, on equivalent areas of the chest wall, that is, over equivalent bronchopulmonary segments, on either side of the chest. Vocal fremitus is most intense in the slender adult male, less intense in women. Increased fremitus on one side indicates that sound is being transmitted better through a more solid, less aerated lung and suggests tissue consolidation, often a result of lobar pneumonia. Decreased or absent fremitus, the result of conditions that favor less sound transmission, may occur when there is fibrous thickening of the pleura, when fluid is present in the pleural space, or when there is air in the pleural space (pneumothorax).

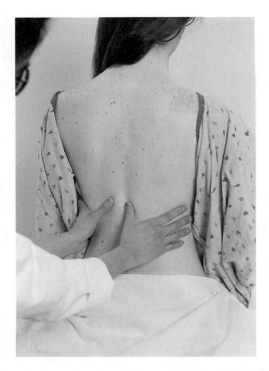

FIGURE 3-11. Respiratory motion of the rib margins. The examiner should watch for the excursion of his or her thumbs and feel for the range and symmetry of respiratory movement. (From Seidel HM, editor: *Mosby's guide to physical examination,* ed 5, St Louis, 2003, Mosby.)

Respiratory motion of the rib margins can be gauged by palpation. The sides of the chest are grasped firmly as in Figure 3-11. The hands should be placed so that there is a loose fold of skin between the two thumbs, which can then move apart as the chest expands. The movement of the thumbs serves as an accurate gauge of the relative movement of the two sides of the chest.

PERCUSSION

Percussion is the tapping of body structures to produce a sound. Two methods of percussion are employed over the chest: (1) *immediate percussion,* during which the examiner strikes the chest with either the palmar aspect of the middle finger or the tips of four fingers held tightly together; and (2) *mediate percussion,* during which the examiner holds a solid object, called the *pleximeter* (commonly the middle finger), against the chest; a second object, the plexor (usually the middle finger of the other hand), strikes the pleximeter, generating a sound (Figures 3-12 and 3-13). As in the evaluation of vocal fremitus, the percussion sound from one side of the

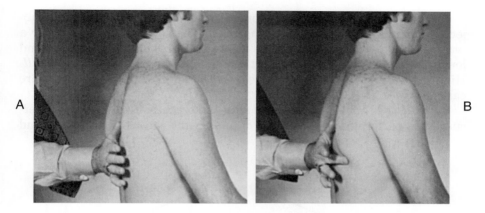

A

B

FIGURE 3-12. Immediate percussion with the middle finger. **A,** The finger posed to strike the chest wall. **B,** The palmar aspect of the finger striking the chest wall. (From Prior JA: Thorax and lungs. In Prior JA, Silberstein JS, Stang JM, editors: *Physical diagnosis,* St Louis, 1981, Mosby.)

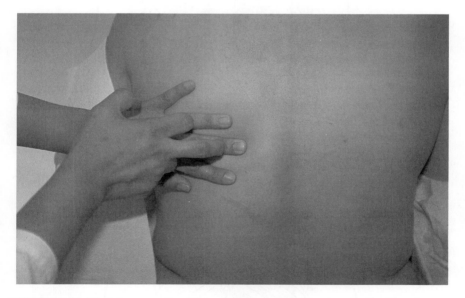

FIGURE 3-13. Mediate percussion. The wrist is cocked and ready to strike. The plexor fingertip is striking the pleximeter finger. Only the pleximeter finger touches the patient's back. (From Lemmi FO, Lemmi CAE: *Physical assessment findings CD-ROM,* Philadelphia, 2000, WB Saunders.)

chest should be compared with the sound on the opposite side. Percussion is generally performed at the following sites: (1) the midportion of each clavicle, (2) the lung apices, (3) the posterior thorax at several points from the apices to the bases of the lungs, (4) the axillary and midaxillary regions, and (5) the anterior portion of the chest (see Figure 4-1).

The percussion sounds vary considerably in quality in different subjects and over different parts of the chest. The sounds generated over a normal lung are often described as *resonant*. Notes of short duration and low intensity, normally found over the liver and the heart, are called *dull*. High-pitched sounds, such as those over the air-containing stomach, are called *tympanitic* (Figure 3-14).

Pathologic changes in the chest alter the percussion sounds. When percussion is performed over an area of pneumonic consolidation, the sound

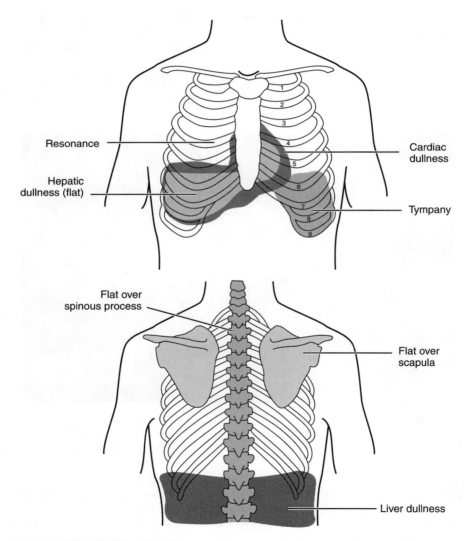

FIGURE 3-14. Regions over the normal thorax where resonance, dullness, and tympany are elicited during percussion.

evoked is dull rather than resonant. Percussion over an emphysematous lung or a pneumothorax produces a deep, sustained *hyperresonant* sound.

Percussion may be used to determine whether position and motion of the diaphragms are normal. First, the patient is told to take a deep breath and hold it. Second, the lower margin of resonance, which represents the level of the diaphragm, is determined by percussion; in doing so, the examiner moves the pleximeter finger downward until a definite change in tonal quality is heard. Third, the patient is instructed to exhale as far as possible and hold his or her breath; percussion is then repeated. The distance between the two levels indicates the range of motion of the diaphragm, normally about 3 to 5 cm (Figure 3-15). The diaphragmatic excursion will be reduced in patients with severe emphysema, pleural inflammation, and splinting because of pain. In carcinoma of the lung, when the phrenic nerve has been damaged, diaphragmatic motion on one side may be absent. In addition, diaphragmatic excursion cannot be assessed in the presence of pleural effusion.

Percussion over the clavicles, a valuable technique in detecting lesions of the upper lobes, differs from that used elsewhere. The clavicles should be percussed directly with the right middle finger or with the right index, middle, and ring fingers held closely together. The medial third of the clavicle, just lateral to its enlarged medial end, yields the best diagnostic information. Percussion more laterally simply elicits dullness from the muscle masses of the shoulder. Auscultation is discussed in Chapter 4.

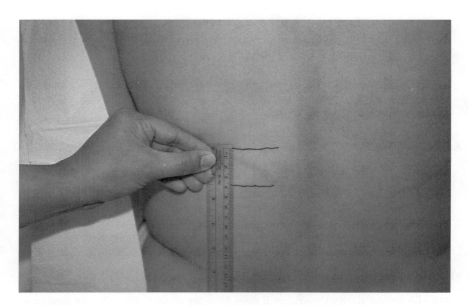

FIGURE 3-15. Normal range of diaphragmatic motion detectable by percussion. (From Lemmi FO, Lemmi CAE: *Physical assessment findings CD-ROM,* Philadelphia, 2000, WB Saunders.)

During ausculatory percussion, the examiner taps his finger gently over the manubrium of the sternum, while listening over the posterior chest wall with a stethoscope. A decrease in sound amplitude is ascribed to a lung abnormality. Some clinicians believe that auscultatory percussion is capable of identifying pulmonary lesions deep within the chest. However, one recent study suggests that the sound of the percussion travels mainly through chest wall structures, not through lung tissue. Therefore, the usefulness of auscultatory percussion in detecting deep chest lesions is highly questionable (Bohadana, Patel, and Kraman, 1989).

CLINICAL AND LABORATORY TESTS
FOR PATHOLOGIC CONDITIONS
Radiographic Examination

Posteroanterior and *lateral radiographs* of the chest may reveal a lesion that was undetected by history and physical examination and show its position, and such radiographs sometimes suggest a pathologic condition. *Chest fluoroscopy* provides information regarding mobility of the diaphragm, which is of particular importance in lung cancer. For example, if one side of the diaphragm is paralyzed, the tumor has probably damaged the phrenic nerve. *Tomography* (Figure 3-16) is a radiographic technique capable of visualizing an opacity or abnormality lying in one particular anatomic plane; the opacity may have been obscured by overlying struc-

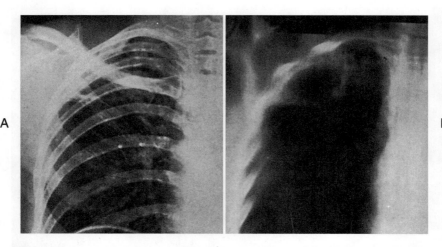

A

B

FIGURE 3-16. Cavity rendered more visible by tomography. **A,** Large cavity in right upper lobe that is barely visible in the routine film. **B,** Tomogram reveals the borders of the cavity with greater clarity. Conventional chest films are made at 2 m, whereas tomograms are made at 1 m or less; there is therefore increased magnification in the latter. (From Hinshaw HC, Murray JF: *Diseases of the chest,* ed 4, Philadelphia, 1980, WB Saunders.)

tures in the ordinary radiograph. Tomography is of particular value in locating lung cavities and flecks of calcium in a lung lesion and in defining irregular densities. *Pulmonary angiography* (Figure 3-17) can be used to differentiate solid chest masses from blood vessels or to detect vascular obstruction. A pulmonary angiogram is made by taking films in quick succession after injecting contrast medium into the main pulmonary artery. *Computerized axial tomography (CT scanning)* employs x-rays and a computer to reconstruct very detailed cross-sectional images. This technique provides an additional dimension to conventional radiography and helps clarify or identify lesions not clearly visualized by other methods.

Radioisotope Scanning

Perfusion scans of the lung are done by intravenously injecting the radioactive compound technetium 99m-labeled microspheres (Figure 3-18). These tiny, biodegradable particles are trapped in the lung tissue. The radiation they emit is collected by a device called a *gamma camera,* which creates an image of the perfused tissue. A second type of scan, a ventilation study, performed by allowing the patient to inhale radioactive xenon gas, can be compared with the perfusion study to diagnose pulmonary embolus (Figure 3-19). For example, if a section of lung is ventilated but

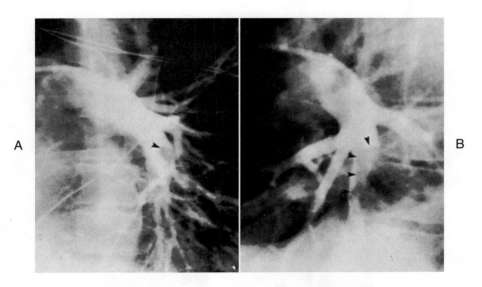

FIGURE 3-17. Selective pulmonary angiography with multiple projections. Angiograms in the anteroposterior projection following injection of dye into the main pulmonary artery were normal. In contrast, angiograms after selective injections into the left main pulmonary artery in the oblique projection **(A)** reveal possible intraluminal filling defect *(arrow);* repeat study in lateral projection **(B)** reveals obvious large embolus *(arrows).* (From Hinshaw HC, Murray JF: *Diseases of the chest,* ed 4, Philadelphia, 1980, WB Saunders.)

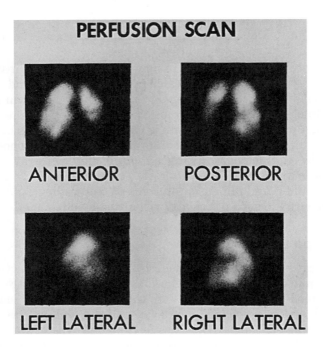

FIGURE 3-18. Perfusion scintiscans. Perfusion lung scan with ^{99m}Tc-albumin of a 49-year-old man, who had been in a long leg cast for 2 weeks and who was complaining of chest pain and dyspnea, showing multiple segmental defects in all four views. Angiography confirmed presence of multiple pulmonary emboli. (From Hinshaw HC, Murray JF: *Diseases of the chest,* ed 4, Philadelphia, 1980, WB Saunders.)

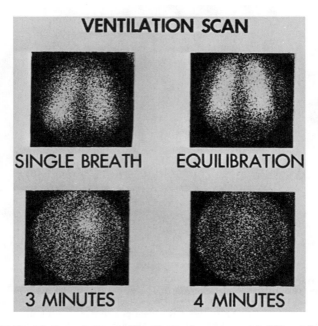

FIGURE 3-19. Ventilation scintiscans. Ventilation lung scan with ^{133}Xe of the same patient described in Figure 3-18, showing even distribution of a single breath of the isotope, uniform labeling of both lungs at equilibration, and nearly even washout at 3 and 4 minutes. (There is slight retention in the right upper lung field.) (From Hinshaw HC, Murray JF: *Diseases of the chest,* ed 4, Philadelphia, 1980, WB Saunders.)

not perfused, an embolus is probably present. But if a section of lung is both unventilated and unperfused, it is probably a bleb- or bulla-containing portion of lung tissue.

Intradermal Tests

The most frequently performed intradermal test is the tuberculin test; a liquid containing the antigen is injected under the skin. If a red wheal forms at the site of injection 24 to 48 hours later, the patient has a present or past infection with tuberculosis. The wheal must be palpable; redness alone is not diagnostic.

Bronchoscopy

The bronchoscope, a rigid tubular instrument, can be inserted through the mouth and the trachea, making examination of the bronchi possible as far as the segmental orifices. A flexible fiberoptic bronchoscope can be inserted considerably farther and can be used to obtain a biopsy of even peripheral lung lesions for definitive diagnosis. In addition, the flexible bronchoscope can be used to obtain pieces of lung tissue from patients with diffuse pulmonary disease (transbronchial biopsy) and to remove secretions or mucous plugs. Bronchoscopy is most often performed when carcinoma is suspected, but it is also used to diagnose an inhaled foreign body as well as other conditions.

Bronchography

In this radiographic technique used to visualize the trachea and bronchi, the bronchial tree is anesthetized with a topical anesthetic, then coated with an oily contrast medium. Bronchography is of value mainly for documenting the presence and extent of bronchiectasis (Figure 3-20).

Mediastinoscopy

During this examination, a rigid tube is inserted into the mediastinum from just above the sternal notch, and any lymph nodes visible can undergo biopsy. This technique is of special value in determining if lung cancer has spread to the mediastinal lymph nodes or if a mediastinal density represents metastatic spread.

Pleural Aspiration and Biopsy

Once the presence of pleural fluid has been documented, a needle may be inserted into the chest to withdraw a sample for laboratory examination.

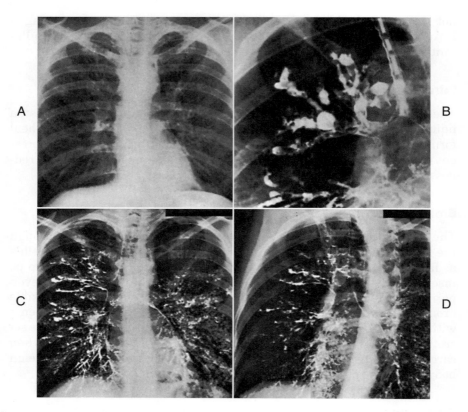

FIGURE 3-20. Bronchography. Chest roentogenogram and three views from subsequent bronchography of a 20-year-old man with chronic cough, intermittent hemoptysis, and foul-smelling sputum. Slight increase in right-sided markings **(A)** is shown to be caused by bronchiectasis of the right and middle lobes **(B, C,** and **D).** (From Hinshaw HC, Murray JF: *Diseases of the chest,* ed 4, Philadelphia, 1980, WB Saunders.)

Pleural biopsy is especially helpful if bacteriologic or pathologic examination reveals the presence of tubercle bacilli or malignant cells.

Oxygen Tension, Carbon Dioxide Tension, and pH

Oxygen tension (PaO_2), carbon dioxide tension ($PaCO_2$), and pH are determined by drawing an arterial blood sample from the radial artery in the wrist, the brachial artery above the elbow, or the femoral artery in the groin. If pulmonary function is poor, PaO_2 is diminished, but $PaCO_2$ may be increased. The pH is diminished as well, indicating that the blood is abnormally acidic, a result of increased hydrogen ion concentration. This condition is referred to as *respiratory acidosis.*

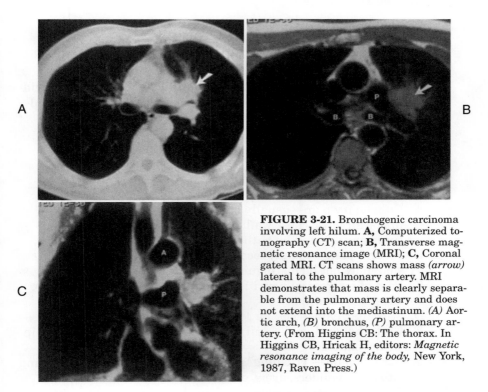

FIGURE 3-21. Bronchogenic carcinoma involving left hilum. **A,** Computerized tomography (CT) scan; **B,** Transverse magnetic resonance image (MRI); **C,** Coronal gated MRI. CT scans shows mass *(arrow)* lateral to the pulmonary artery. MRI demonstrates that mass is clearly separable from the pulmonary artery and does not extend into the mediastinum. *(A)* Aortic arch, *(B)* bronchus, *(P)* pulmonary artery. (From Higgins CB: The thorax. In Higgins CB, Hricak H, editors: *Magnetic resonance imaging of the body,* New York, 1987, Raven Press.)

Magnetic Resonance Imaging

Magnetic resonance imaging (MRI) uses a powerful magnet and a computer to create images of body structures. MRI images of the chest show greater contrast between lesions and blood vessels than do CT scans (Figure 3-21).

SUMMARY OF THE HISTORY AND PHYSICAL EXAMINATION

History

  I. Chief complaint—Why has the patient come for medical help?
 II. Family and social history
    A. History of tuberculosis?
    B. History of allergic disorder or asthma?
    C. Environmental air pollution?
    D. Cigarette smoking (evaluated in pack-years = packs per day × number of years smoked)

III. Occupational history
  A. Exposure to industrial dusts—silica, asbestos?
  B. Exposure to pigeons, parrots, or parakeets? Psittacosis may result
  C. Residence in California's San Joaquin Valley? Consider coccidioidomycosis; histoplasmosis in patients from eastern or midwestern United States
IV. History of previous illness
  A. Tuberculosis
  B. Pneumonia or "pleurisy"
  C. Chest injuries and operations
V. Pain
  A. Pulmonary pain—usually occurs when the parietal pleura, major airways, chest wall, diaphragm, or mediastinal structures are affected by pathologic processes
  B. Pleural pain—usually localized, aggravated by chest expansion, may not be distinguishable from pulmonary pain
  C. Pain of intercostal neuritis—superficial, related to coughing, sneezing, straining
  D. Muscular pain—look for local tenderness to palpation
  E. Costochondral pain—dull, gnawing, aching, little relationship to movement
  F. Cardiac pain—"crushing" pain beneath the sternum, radiating into the shoulders, arms, or neck
  G. Pericardial pain—similar to pleural pain, relieved by sitting up and leaning forward
  H. Aortic pain—especially of a dissecting aneurysm, described as substernal, deep, boring, agonizing, tearing
  I. Pulmonary embolus—chest pain associated with shortness of breath, rarely hemoptysis, cough
VI. Cough
  A. Suggests abnormality when persistent
  B. Two types of cough
    1. Productive—clears airways of secretions
    2. Nonproductive—irritative, serves no useful purpose ("dry cough")
  C. Type of sputum suggests pathologic process
    1. Foul smelling—lung abscess
    2. Abundant, frothy, saliva-like—bronchoalveolar carcinoma
    3. Voluminous, pink, frothy—pulmonary edema
    4. Rust-colored—pneumococcal pneumonia
    5. Copious, purulent, brought up with posture change—bronchiectasis
VII. Hemoptysis—coughing up blood
  A. Most patients with hemoptysis have bronchitis, but some may be seriously ill

    B. Blood from gastrointestinal tract (hematemesis) or nasopharynx may be confused with blood from the lung

VIII. Dyspnea—shortness of breath or difficulty breathing

    A. Ask circumstances—association with climbing two flights of steps or walking a half block?

    B. Dyspnea is occasionally psychogenic or emotional

IX. Hoarseness

    A. Usually an abnormality of vocal cords

    B. May be the result of lung tumor or aortic aneurysm damage of recurrent laryngeal nerve

X. Wheeze—a musical sound described fully in Chapter 5

Physical Examination

I. Inspection—general

    A. Evaluate breathlessness, wheezing, sputum, and cough

    B. Observe skin for cyanosis and pallor, eruptions, nodules, scars

    C. Look for neck vein distention

    D. Examine fingers for tobacco stains, fingers and toes for clubbing

    E. Evaluate anteroposterior diameter relative to lateral diameter of chest wall

    F. Look for pectus carinatum ("pigeon breast"), pectus excavatum ("funnel chest"), kyphosis (abnormally increased spine curvature), scoliosis (lateral spine curvature), kyphoscoliosis

    G. Observe tracheal position; it should be midline

II. Inspection—respiratory motions

    A. Note whether chest expansion is bilaterally symmetric

    B. Look for abnormal breathing

      1. Bradypnea—abnormally slow breathing

      2. Tachypnea—abnormally fast breathing

      3. Apnea—temporary cessation of respiration

      4. Hyperpnea—increase in depth of breathing ("air hunger")

      5. Periodic respiration—alternating hyperpnea and apnea

      6. Sighing respiration, deep breaths interrupting normal rhythm, is commonly a sign of emotional tension

    C. Note mode of breathing—thoracic or abdominal

III. Palpation

    A. Examine neck, axillae, and supraclavicular fossae for lymph nodes; biopsy of these may be the only practical means of diagnosing lung cancer

    B. Palpate trachea to detect any deviation from the midline, or deviation anteriorly

    C. Palpate chest wall while patient says "one, two, three" or "ninety-nine" to detect increased or decreased vibrations (vocal or tactile fremitus)

    D. Gauge respiratory motions of the rib margins to assess relative movement of the two sides of the chest

IV. Percussion—tapping body structures to produce a sound

    A. Percussion sounds from similar areas on each side of the chest should be compared

    B. Percuss to determine whether diaphragmatic motion is normal

V. Auscultation—see Chapter 4

Chapter Review and Critical Thinking Questions

1. *What are the elements of the chief complaint?*

2. *Why is occupational history important?*

3. *About which previous illnesses should the caregiver specifically inquire?*

4. *What are two types of cough?*

5. *What two pulmonary diseases are commonly associated with massive hemoptysis?*

BIBLIOGRAPHY

Bates BA: *A guide to physical examination,* Philadelphia, 1974, JB Lippincott.

Bohadana AB, Patel R, Kraman SS: Contour maps of auscultatory percussion in healthy subjects and patients with large intrapulmonary lesions, *Lung* 167:359-372, 1989.

Delp MH, Manning RT: *Major's physical diagnosis,* Philadelphia, 1980, WB Saunders.

Forgacs P: *Lung sounds,* London, 1978, Bailliere Tindall.

Grant I: The respiratory system. In Macleod J, editor: *Clinical examination,* Edinburgh, 1979, Churchill Livingstone.

Higgins CB: The thorax. In CB Higgins, Hricak HH, editors: *Magnetic resonance imaging of the body,* New York, 1987, Raven Press.

Hinshaw HC, Murray JF: *Diseases of the chest,* ed 4, Philadelphia, 1980, WB Saunders.

Naidich D, Zerhouni EA, Siegelman SS: *Computed tomography of the thorax,* New York, 1984, Raven Press.

Prior JA, Silberstein JS: *Physical diagnosis,* ed 6, St Louis, 1981, Mosby.

Rabin C: New or neglected signs in the diagnosis of chest disease. In Fishman AP, editor: *Pulmonary diseases and disorders,* New York, 1980, McGraw-Hill.

Thrope CW, Fright WR, Toop LJ et al: A microcomputer-based interactive cough sound analysis system, *Comput Methods Programs Biomed* 36:33-43, 1991.

Chapter 4

Normal Breath Sounds

How are the normal sounds of breathing produced? This question has puzzled investigators since the beginning of the nineteenth century. Researchers now believe that these normal sounds are produced by the turbulent flow of air in the lobar and segmental bronchi. No sounds are produced by air moving in and out of the alveoli because the airflow here is slower and probably nonturbulent.

This chapter discusses normal breath sounds by presenting the following topics:

1. Auscultation.
2. Early experiments. One erroneously led to the conclusion that normal breath sounds are produced in the alveoli.
3. Turbulence and breath sounds. Rapidly flowing air moves in a noisy, turbulent manner; slowly flowing air moves in a silent, laminar manner. Because airflow is most turbulent in the trachea and the first few generations of bronchi, normal breath sounds are most likely produced here.
4. Regional airflow and breath sounds. Studies of the lung have shown that there are regional differences in sound intensity at the apex and base of the lung. These fluctuations reflect differences that have been measured in regional airflow.
5. Variation of breath sounds with the heartbeat. Breath sounds over the left lower lobe of the lung become louder when the heart contracts and the adjacent lung tissue expands, lowering alveolar pressure and facilitating airflow into the left lower lobe. This observation again confirms the relationship of airflow to production of breath sounds.
6. Breath sounds at the mouth.
7. Breath sounds over the chest and trachea.
8. Phonopneumography. This technique allows the visual display of breath sounds. It has been used both for teaching and for breath sounds research, showing, for example, that the loudest point on the chest wall is the area immediately below the clavicle anteriorly.

The field of breath sounds research has expanded greatly in the last few years; much of the recent work is described in this chapter, and it provides background and understanding for anyone who wishes to follow new developments as they occur.

AUSCULTATION

With the patient sitting upright, comparative auscultation of the region overlying each pulmonary segment should be made. The stethoscope should be moved back and forth between comparable pulmonary segments on either side of the chest (Figure 4-1). Auscultation should not be performed by moving the stethoscope down one side and then down the other. Each region should be listened to carefully while the patient is breathing through the mouth at a slightly increased rate and depth.

The examiner should first concentrate on inspiration—its length and its normal and adventitial components (crackles, wheezes, and so on; see

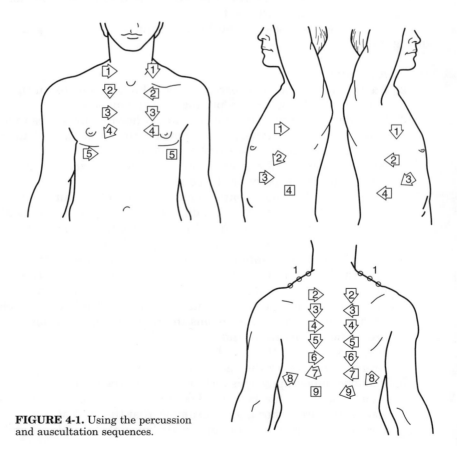

FIGURE 4-1. Using the percussion and auscultation sequences.

Chapter 5). The examiner should then note the same phenomena in expiration.

The chest should always be auscultated in a quiet room. Radios and television sets should be turned off. The examiner should try to avoid listening over chest hair. When the hair moves against the diaphragm of the stethoscope during breathing, a crackling (adventitious) sound is produced that is quite similar to that heard within the lungs in certain pathologic conditions; when unavoidable, wetting the hair reduces or prevents this phenomenon. The stethoscope should not be used over clothing because the breath sounds are then difficult to hear. The tubing should not touch clothing, bedsheets, or other objects, because this produces artifactual noise.

Four types of breath sounds are heard over the normal chest (Figures 4-2 and 4-3):

1. *Normal vesicular.* This is a relatively soft, low-pitched sound, sometimes described as a sighing or gentle rustling; it is heard over most of the peripheral parts of the lung. The inspiratory (I) phase is markedly longer than the expiratory phase (E), with the I:E ratio being about 3:1. Expiration is much quieter than inspiration, usually being almost inaudible. There is no pause between inspiration and expiration.

    The term *vesicular* is a misnomer. As is discussed more fully later, the term came from experiments performed in the nineteenth century suggesting that the normal sounds arose in the alveoli, then called "vesicles." In fact, modern engineering concepts make it more likely that these sounds emanate from the turbulent flow of air in the lobar and segmental bronchi, not the alveoli.

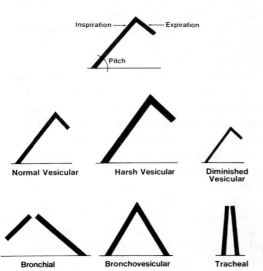

FIGURE 4-2. Diagrammatic representation of normal breath sounds.

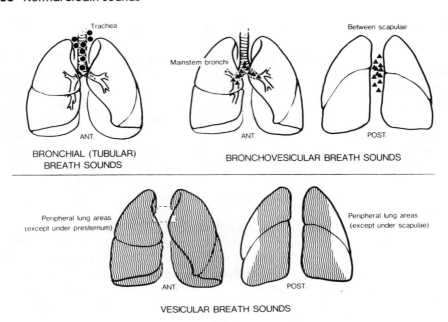

FIGURE 4-3. Breath sounds over the normal chest.

2. *Bronchial.* These characteristically loud, high-pitched sounds resemble the sound of air blowing through a hollow pipe. Their expiratory phase is louder and longer than their inspiratory phase. They are normally present only over the manubrium, and a distinct pause can be heard between the inspiratory and expiratory phases. The appearance of bronchial sounds over the periphery of the lung may mean abnormal sound transmission because of consolidated lung tissue, as in pneumonia or atelectasis. This phenomenon is discussed in Chapter 5.

3. *Bronchovesicular.* These sounds are a mixture of bronchial and vesicular sounds. Their inspiratory and expiratory phases are about equal in length (I:E ratio = 1:1). They are normally audible in two places: (1) anteriorly, near the mainstem bronchi in the first and second intercostal spaces; and (2) posteriorly, between the scapulae. To hear them elsewhere may mean lung consolidation or another abnormality.

4. *Tracheal.* These sounds, not usually auscultated, are present over the extrathoracic portion of the trachea. They are very loud, very high-pitched, and have a hollow or harsh quality. The expiratory phase is slightly longer than the inspiratory phase.

I:E ratios of tracheal and bronchial sounds are about the same. The major determinant of the length of the expiratory

TABLE 4-1. Physical Findings in Some Common Pulmonary Disorders

Disorder	Inspection	Palpation	Percussion	Auscultation
Bronchial asthma (acute attack)	Hyperinflation Use of accessory muscles	Impaired expansion Decreased fremitus	Hyperresonance Low diaphragms	Prolonged expiration Wheezes
Pneumothorax (complete)	Lag on affected side	Absent fremitus	Hyperresonant or tympanitic	Absent breath sounds
Pleural effusion (large)	Lag on affected side	Decreased fremitus Trachea and heart shifted away from affected side	Dullness or flatness	Absent breath sounds
Atelectasis (lobar obstruction)	Lag on affected side	Decreased fremitus Trachea and heart shifted toward affected side	Dullness or flatness	Absent breath sounds
Consolidation (pneumonia)	Possible lag or splinting on affected side	Increased fremitus	Dullness	Bronchial breath sounds Bronchophony Pectoriloquy

From Hinshaw HC, Murray JF: *Diseases of the chest*, ed 4, Philadelphia, 1980, WB Saunders.

sound is its loudness. At the lung bases, only the loudest portion of the sound can be heard; therefore it seems short.

Physical findings in some common pulmonary disorders are presented in Table 4-1.

EARLY EXPERIMENTS

In 1819 Rene Theophile Laennec recorded the first description of the normal lung sound: "A slight but extremely distinct murmur answering to the entrance of air into and its expulsion from the air cells of the lung." At the time, no one was certain whether this sound was produced within the larynx or within the lungs themselves (Laennec, 1935; Murphy, 1981).

In 1884 J. F. Bullar, an English surgeon, made the first effort to elucidate the correct mechanism (Bullar, 1884). He constructed an artificial thorax made of an airtight, fluid-filled chamber with glass sides, which could be expanded and contracted with a bellows (Figure 4-4). Within the artificial thorax he placed one of two sheep lungs, connected to the other (which was left outside) by its trachea and bronchi. Even when the trachea was plugged, he found that he could produce normal breath sounds.

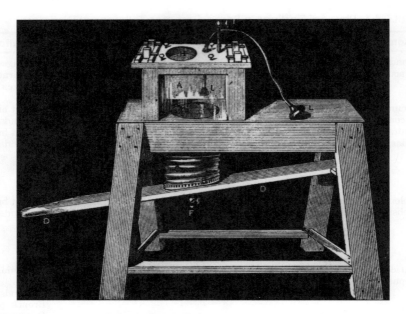

FIGURE 4-4. In 1884 J. F. Bullar, an English surgeon, used this artificial thorax to investigate the origin of breath sounds. (From Bullar JF: *Proc R Soc Lond* 37:411-423, 1884.)

Bullar concluded correctly that these normal sounds were produced within the lungs but incorrectly surmised that they were generated as air passed from the terminal bronchioles into the alveoli. Years later, an American investigator, R. R. Hannon, performed other experiments confirming Bullar's observation that some normal sounds are produced in the lung (Hannon and Lyman, 1929).

TURBULENCE AND BREATH SOUNDS

Turbulence in the airstream is believed to be the source of normal breath sounds (Forgacs, 1978). To appreciate this fact fully, one should have some knowledge of the three types of fluid flow: (1) laminar flow, (2) turbulent flow, and (3) vortices.

Laminar Flow

When a fluid, such as air, is flowing slowly along a straight, smooth pipe, it flows in streamlines or layers parallel with the walls of the pipe. The pressure driving the fluid is gradually dissipated by forces that occur between neighboring streamlines and between the gas and the walls of the pipe. Because there are no sudden changes or oscillations of pressure, no sound waves are generated.

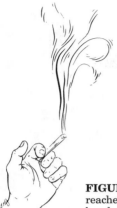

FIGURE 4-5. Turbulent flow and laminar flow. When the flow of a fluid reaches a critical velocity, the orderly arrangement of the streamlines breaks up, and small packets of gas begin to move at random across or against the general direction of flow.

Turbulent Flow

When the fluid flow reaches a critical velocity, the orderly arrangement of the streamlines breaks up, and small packets of gas begin to move at random across or against the general direction of flow. A common example of laminar and turbulent flow is the stream of smoke emanating from a lit cigarette (Figure 4-5). Close to the cigarette, the flow is laminar, that is, smooth and regular. Farther away, the flow becomes more disorderly, that is, turbulent.

In turbulent flow, energy is transferred between colliding packets of gas, and transient pressure variations occur, generating sound. The noise produced by these rapid gas fluctuations varies at random in amplitude, with an even frequency distribution between 200 and 2000 Hz, or approximately the frequencies of normal speech. By analogy with the frequency spectrum of white light, such sound is often described as *white noise*.

Turbulence begins at a critical flow velocity. From experimental observations of gas flow and by calculation, investigators have learned that airflow is turbulent in the trachea and the first few generations of bronchi. In the peripheral bronchi, the slower flow becomes laminar and silent. Between these two regions an intermediate zone exists, extending from the segmental bronchi to the fifteenth generation of the airways. Here the laminar flow pattern is disrupted by vortices.

Vortices

When a stream of gas emerges from a slit or circular orifice into a wider channel, the forces arising at the boundary between the stream and the surrounding fluid generate whirlpools, or vortices. Vortices are also pro-

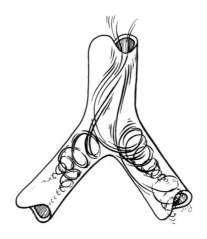

FIGURE 4-6. Vortices. When a stream of gas emerges from a slit or circular orifice into a wider channel, the forces arising at the boundary between the stream and the surrounding fluid generate whirlpools or vortices.

duced when a curvature or angle in the pipe forces flow to change direction abruptly. These conditions cause the gas stream to separate into layers that move forward at different velocities. The slower streams are turned into circular motion by the force of the high-velocity streams flowing alongside (Figure 4-6). The resulting noise has a wide frequency spectrum, the lower frequencies probably being more prominent in the periphery of the lung.

Two observations support the view that high airflow rate, vortices, and turbulence produce breath sounds in the larger airways: (1) the relationship between regional airflow rate and breath sounds, and (2) the variation with the heartbeat of the breath sounds over the left lower lobe of the lung.

REGIONAL AIRFLOW AND BREATH SOUNDS

Measurements of inspiratory breath sounds through the chest wall show that there are regional differences in sound intensity at the apex and base of the lung (Leblanc, Macklem, and Ross, 1970; Ploysongsang, Martin, Ross et al., 1977; Shykoff, Ploysongsang, and Chang, 1988).

In a normal individual in the upright position, breath sounds at the apex become progressively fainter during inspiration from residual volume. In contrast, at the base, the breath sounds are relatively faint at the beginning of inspiration; their intensity increases to a maximum at 50% of the vital capacity (Figure 4-7). These fluctuations reflect differences that have been measured in regional airflow rates. In the apex, airflow begins immediately, regardless of the initial lung volume. At the base, the inspiratory airflow does not begin until the dependent airways, which are normally closed at low lung volumes, reopen.

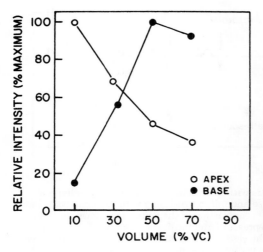

FIGURE 4-7. Relative intensity of breath sounds plotted against lung volume (as percentage of vital capacity) in one subject. Note that the breath sounds at the apex become progressively fainter during inspiration. In contrast, at the base, the breath sounds are relatively faint at the beginning of inspiration, and their intensity increases to a maximum at 50% of the vital capacity. These results correlated well with the differences in regional distribution of ventilation found with radioactive gases. (From Leblanc P, Macklem PT, Ross WRD: *Am Rev Respir Dis* 102:1016, 1970.)

In addition, breath sounds over the anterior upper chest are louder on the right than on the left. At the posterior lung base, breath sounds are louder on the left. The asymmetry is probably related to the effects of cardiovascular structures and airway geometry on sound generation and transmission (Pasterkamp, Patel, Wodicka, 1997).

VARIATION OF BREATH SOUNDS

Breath Sounds with Heartbeat

In some healthy individuals, breath sounds over the left lower lobe rise and fall in synchrony with the heartbeat. Usually, they are loudest during systole, when contraction of the ventricles allows the adjacent lung tissue to expand, lowering alveolar pressure and facilitating gas flow into the left lower lobe. Simultaneous recordings of the electrocardiogram and the breath sounds over the left lower lobe verify that the sounds become more intense at the R wave and reach their peak at the T wave (Figure 4-8). This peak may be as much as 40% above the mean. Interestingly, in some persons, an opposite effect is associated with the heartbeat: The breath sounds become quieter during ventricular systole. Apparently, the movement of the heart into the left lower lobe has compressed the lung and transiently reduced the regional airflow rate.

Breath Sounds at the Mouth

Breath sounds at the mouth are different from sounds heard through the chest wall because of different paths of transmission. In large tubes, such as the trachea and main bronchi, sound travels well and reaches the

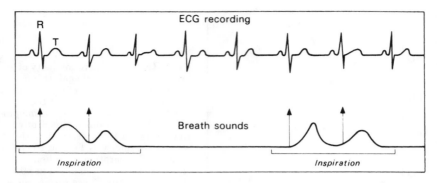

FIGURE 4-8. Variations of breath sounds with heartbeat. In some healthy individuals, breath sounds over the left lower lobe rise and fall in synchrony with the heartbeat. Usually, they are loudest during systole, when contraction of the ventricles allows the adjacent lung tissue to expand, lowering gas pressure and facilitating gas flow into the left lower lobe. Simultaneous recordings of the electrocardiogram and the breath sounds over the left lower lobe verify that the sounds become more intense at the R wave and reach their peak at the T wave. (From Forgacs P: *Lung sounds,* London, 1978, Baillière Tindall.)

mouth almost unfiltered. However, sounds that must travel through the lung and chest wall are filtered; they fall into a relatively narrow range of low frequencies, with a steep fall in amplitude above 200 Hz. In contrast, the breath sounds at the mouth consist of a broad range of evenly distributed frequencies between 200 and 2000 cycles (Figure 4-9). In other words, the chest wall and lung are acting as a so-called low pass filter and are allowing only the low frequencies to pass through.

Breath Sounds over the Chest and Trachea

Breath sounds transmitted through the chest fade out during expiration, whereas those over the trachea can be heard throughout the respiratory cycle. There are at least two reasons for this:

1. Although rate of airflow falls continuously during expiration, the breath sounds over the trachea are so loud that they remain above the threshold of hearing throughout the respiratory cycle. The sounds transmitted through the chest wall are much fainter, and they contain mostly low frequencies, to which the ear is less sensitive. Thus the breath sounds become too soft to hear early in expiration.
2. During inspiration, turbulence is most likely generated and carried farther toward the periphery of the lung than during expiration. Because the turbulence moves away from the chest wall during expiration, the resulting faint breath sounds are absorbed by the lung before they reach the stethoscope.

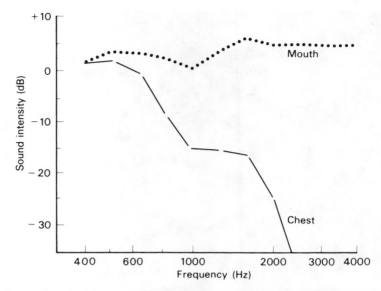

FIGURE 4-9. Intensity and frequency of breath sounds transmitted through the mouth and the chest. Note that the sounds traveling through the chest wall and lung are filtered, falling into a relatively narrow range of low frequencies with a steep fall in amplitude above 200 Hz. In contrast, the breath sounds at the mouth consist of a broad range of evenly distributed frequencies between 200 and 2000 Hz. (From Forgacs P: *Lung sounds,* London, 1978, Baillière Tindall.)

Breath Sounds in Children

Clinicians who auscultate the chest of normal children note that the sound quality varies with age. In fact, studies of the amplitude-frequency spectrum of the sounds confirm that there is a change with age of the frequency content. The breath sounds of very young children have more high frequency components than do those of adults; therefore, they sound higher pitched (Kanga and Kraman, 1986; Hidalgo, Wegman, and Waring, 1991).

PHONOPNEUMOGRAPHY

Phonopneumograms, which are visual displays of breath sounds, are used both as an analytic research device and as a clinical teaching tool. They are useful research tools because a visual plot of a breath sound can be analyzed in considerably more detail than can the same sound heard through a stethoscope. As a teaching device, phonopneumograms can present slowly and clearly to the eye a sound pattern that to the ear might be transient and difficult to interpret.

Some of the most informative early phonopneumograms were recorded by Dr. Victor A. McKusick in 1955 (Figures 4-10 and 4-11). McKusick used a special device called a *sound spectrograph* and made

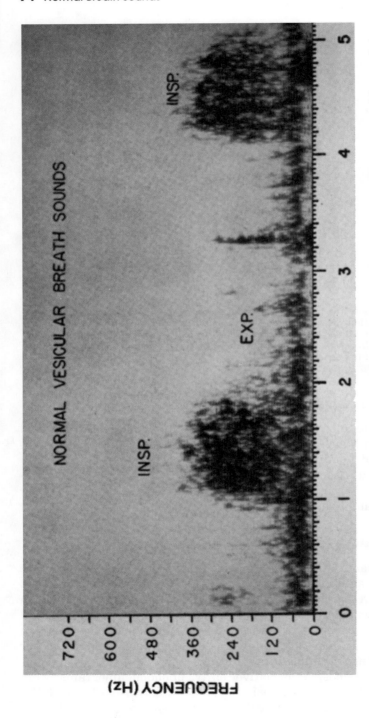

FIGURE 4-10. Sound spectrogram of normal vesicular breath sounds made by Dr. Victor McKusick in 1955. The intensity of the sounds is represented by the darkness of the patterns in the tracing. Note that inspiration is louder and higher pitched than expiration. (From McKusick VA, Jenkins WT, Webb GN: *Am Rev Tuberc* 72:12-34, 1955.)

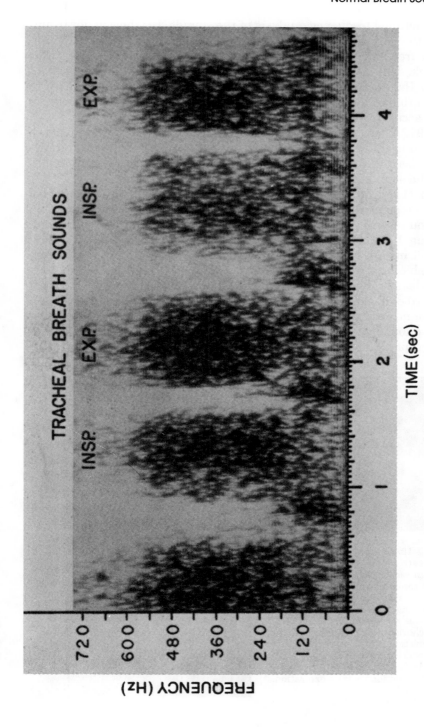

FIGURE 4-11. Tracheal breath sounds recorded by Dr. Victor McKusick on the sound spectrograph. Note that inspiration and expiration are about the same pitch. (From McKusick VA, Jenkins WT, Webb GN: *Am Rev Tuberc* 72:12-34, 1955.)

the first detailed frequency analysis of the sounds. He showed, for example, that the normal inspiratory vesicular sounds were of maximal intensity at a frequency of about 200 Hz and decreased rapidly thereafter (McKusick, Jenkins, and Webb, 1955). He found no sound energy at more than 500 Hz. As noted in Chapter 2, the ear is relatively insensitive to sounds in this frequency range; thus, breath sounds are more difficult to perceive accurately than is normal speech.

In 1972 Weiss and Carlson published calibrated amplitude plots of breath sounds that were recorded on tape and then fed into an oscilloscope (Weiss and Carlson, 1972). These plots revealed the overall amplitude of the sounds during inspiration and expiration (Figure 4-12).

In 1971 Dr. David W. Cugell of the Northwestern University School of Medicine pointed out the importance of both phonopneumograms and breath sound recordings in teaching chest auscultation to medical students (Cugell, 1971). He prepared a questionnaire to determine the level of interest in tape recordings of breath sounds and found that although considerable interest existed, little use was made of audiovisual materials. The dearth of such material at the time prompted Dr. Cugell to test and describe an admirable system for making phonopneumograms and breath sound recordings.

The phonopneumogram is especially useful if it is displayed with a plotted graph that simultaneously shows the precise phase of inspiration

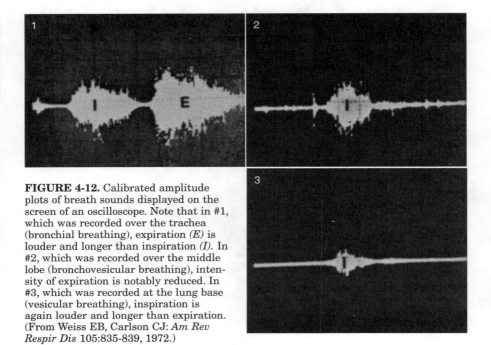

FIGURE 4-12. Calibrated amplitude plots of breath sounds displayed on the screen of an oscilloscope. Note that in #1, which was recorded over the trachea (bronchial breathing), expiration *(E)* is louder and longer than inspiration *(I)*. In #2, which was recorded over the middle lobe (bronchovesicular breathing), intensity of expiration is notably reduced. In #3, which was recorded at the lung base (vesicular breathing), inspiration is again louder and longer than expiration. (From Weiss EB, Carlson CJ: *Am Rev Respir Dis* 105:835-839, 1972.)

or expiration (Banaszak, Kory, and Snider, 1973). This double display is accomplished by adding a device called a *pneumotachometer* to create the phase chart and display the velocity of breathing. The apparatus for making the entire recording is shown in Figure 4-13, and a typical recording is shown in Figure 4-14.

RECORDING SYSTEM

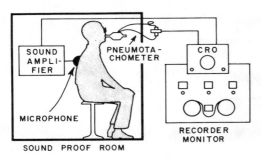

DATA ANALYSIS SYSTEM

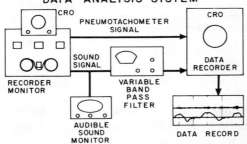

FIGURE 4-13. System for simultaneous recording of breath sounds and breathing velocity. *CRO,* Cathode ray oscilloscope. (From Banaszak EF, Kory RIC, Snider GL: *Am Rev Respir Dis* 107:449-455, 1973.)

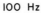

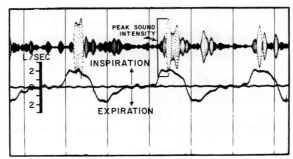

FIGURE 4-14. Typical recording made with the system shown in Figure 4-13. The system is set up to be most sensitive to sounds at 100 Hz. Sound intensity is represented by the upper tracing, flow rate by the lower tracing. (From Banaszak EF, Kory RIC, Snider GL: *Am Rev Respir Dis* 107:449-455, 1973.)

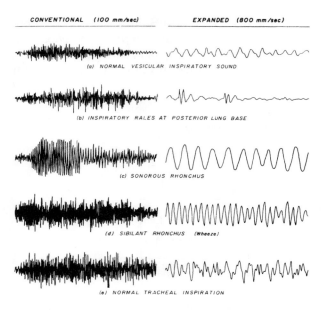

FIGURE 4-15. Amplitude versus time plots of typical lung sounds, showing that the expanded time scales in the right column reveal visually distinct patterns that are not well seen in conventional plots. Time is on the horizontal axis and amplitude is on the vertical axis. The effective chart recorder speeds are 100 mm/sec and 800 mm/sec. (From Murphy RLH, Holford SK, Knowler WC: *N Engl J Med* 296:968-971, 1977.)

A drawback to the phonopneumogram just presented is that normal lung sounds cannot be visually distinguished from abnormal or adventitious sounds, such as crackles and wheezes. Their frequency is simply too high. To circumvent this problem, Dr. Raymond L. Murphy, Jr. used a technique known as time-expanded waveform analysis (Murphy, Holford, and Knowler, 1977). After storing the recorded sounds in the memory of a computer, he replayed the signal at a much slower rate. These time-expanded waveforms of typical sounds showed patterns that allowed the various categories of sound to be visually distinguished from one another (Figure 4-15). In addition, artifactual sounds could be distinguished from true lung sounds (Figure 4-16).

Dr. Steve S. Kraman has made innovative use of phonopneumography. Dr. Kraman has employed a technique, subtraction phonopneumography, to determine the site of production of respiratory sounds (Kraman, 1980).

In subtraction phonopneumography, simultaneous recordings of the lung sounds are made from two different areas of the chest. These recordings are then analyzed to determine whether they represent (1) the same or a similar sound transmitted to each microphone from one or more dis-

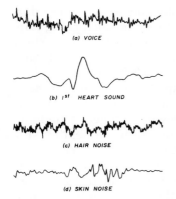

(a) VOICE

(b) 1ˢᵗ HEART SOUND

(c) HAIR NOISE

(d) SKIN NOISE

FIGURE 4-16. Artifactual sounds displayed as time-expanded waveforms have different patterns from the lung sounds shown in Figure 4-15. **A,** Voice sounds recorded with the microphone on the subject's chest. **B,** The first heart sound recorded on the left anterior part of the chest. **C,** Vesicular sounds with superimposed noise of the microphone moving over chest hair. **D,** A plot resulting from sliding the microphone across the skin. (From Murphy RLH, Holford SK, Knowler WC: *N Engl J Med* 296:968-971,1977.)

tant sources, or (2) dissimilar sounds transmitted from sources located near each microphone. Because the normal sounds of breathing are well heard over virtually all of the chest surface, one may assume that a single, centrally produced sound would be transmitted through the lung to the periphery and would arrive in an identical form (in phase) at two different locations on the chest wall that are equidistant from the source. However, a peripherally produced sound, that is, a sound emanating from the subpleural alveolar sacs, would sound loudest to the microphone under which it was produced and would be different from a peripherally produced sound generated directly under the second microphone; in other words, the two sounds would be dissimilar in phase. Thus if one sound is electronically subtracted from another, two similar sounds in phase will cancel each other out, whereas two dissimilar sounds will not.

During this experiment, Dr. Kraman found that when the microphones were placed 4 cm apart, normal persons had at least 50% cancellation of the normal inspiratory sound. In contrast, in recordings of pleural friction rubs, there was no cancellation with microphones placed over opposite lungs. As a result, he concluded that the source of the main component of the normal inspiratory sound is more peripheral than the mainstem bronchi but farther from the chest wall than the pleura—how far is impossible to tell.

Dr. Kraman found that expiratory sounds come from a more central location than inspiratory sounds. In fact, some of the sound seemed to be emanating from above the point, the carina, where the trachea bifurcates into the two mainstem bronchi. Because students are commonly taught that sounds from the larynx are transmitted to the periphery and form part of the normal vesicular breath sounds (Bushnell, 1921), Dr. Kraman designed a second experiment to test the validity of this notion (Kraman, 1981).

The study was designed around the hypothesis that if the laryngeal noise forms an audible part of the vesicular sound heard on the chest wall during quiet breathing, then the vesicular sound should get louder during voluntarily produced noisy breathing. However, no such thing happened. Sounds were recorded from the larynx and four sites on the chest wall simultaneously during quiet breathing and during voluntarily produced noisy breathing. Despite several-fold increases in the amplitude of the laryngeal noise in both inspiration and expiration, the amplitude of the simultaneously recorded vesicular sound correlated only with flow rates and was completely unaffected by changes in laryngeal sound amplitude (Figure 4-17). Therefore during quiet breathing in healthy subjects, no detectable component of the laryngeal noise is likely to reach the periphery.

Dr. Dennis O'Donnell and Dr. Kraman, using automated phonopneumography, have also attempted to document the relative intensity patterns of lung sounds on the chest wall. By employing computerized analysis, they were able to record more than 50 positions on each side of the chest wall in eight normal subjects within a relatively short time. They found that, in general, the loudest point on the chest wall is the area im-

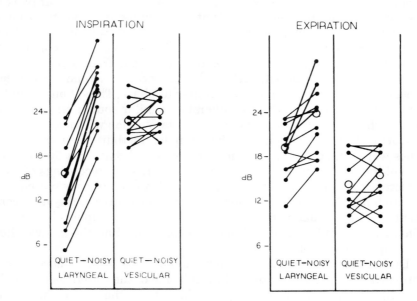

FIGURE 4-17. Relative amplitude of quiet and noisy breaths recorded from the larynx and four positions on the chest wall. The closed circles represent the intensity of each breath. The open circles represent the mean intensity of 12 breaths. Note that over the larynx during inspiration, the noisy breaths are significantly louder than the quiet breaths, whereas over the chest wall (vesicular) there is no significant difference between the amplitudes of the quiet and noisy breaths. The situation is similar in expiration. These findings demonstrate that during quiet breathing in healthy subjects, no detectable laryngeal noise can be heard in the vesicular breath sounds. (From Kraman S: *Am Rev Respir Dis* 124:292-294, 1981.)

mediately below the clavicle anteriorly. Furthermore, chest wall thickness is not a major determinant of the amplitude of the vesicular sounds recorded on the surface of the chest. These sounds are distributed in an irregular succession of sound hills and valleys, with the loudest areas at the apices and bases (Figure 4-18). The right or left lung sound intensities, although proportional to airflow at any one site, may vary by a considerable degree when compared with equally ventilated corresponding areas over the opposite lung (O'Donnell and Kraman, 1982), although the sound intensity at the left apex is always louder than or equal to that at the right (Kraman, 1983) and is linearly associated with airflow (Kraman, 1984). The finding of sound hills and valleys is most surprising because many researchers had believed that lung sound intensity was relatively uniform over the chest of normal subjects (Dosani and Kraman, 1983).

Phonopneumographic Monitoring During Intubation

A practical application of phonopneumography, now in the experimental stages, is the monitoring of patients undergoing general anesthesia. Although mortality related to anesthesia is low, incorrect placement of the endotracheal tube during intubation is still a hazard. Huang, Kraman,

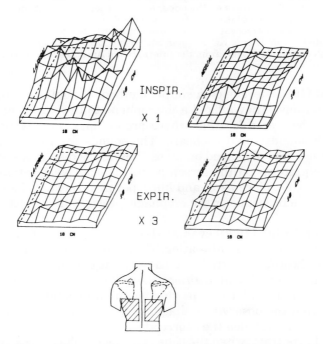

FIGURE 4-18. Three-dimensional sound contour map of a single subject. Note that the sound is distributed in an irregular succession of hills and valleys over the chest wall. (From Dosani R, Kraman SS: *Chest* 83:628-631, 1983.)

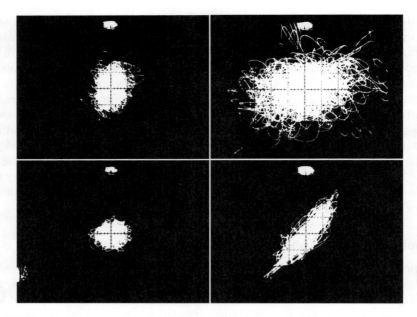

FIGURE 4-19. Lung sound patterns of patients undergoing anesthesia displayed on an oscilloscope screen. The pictures on the upper and lower left show that the endotracheal tube is properly placed, ventilating the trachea. The pictures on the upper and lower right show that the endotracheal tube has been improperly placed, and the esophagus is being ventilated. (From Huang KC, Kraman SS, Wright BD: *Anesth Analg* 62:586-589, 1983. Reprinted with permission from the International Anesthesia Research Society.)

and Wright (1983) developed a simple method of monitoring the ventilation of both lungs. They affixed a microphone to the skin overlying each side of the chest at a location where preliminary auscultation showed that breath sounds could be heard. The sounds from each microphone were amplified and displayed on an oscilloscope screen in a so-called X-Y format. The patterns on the screen permitted easy verification of proper endotracheal tube placement, and improper placement of the tube in the right mainstem bronchus or the esophagus was readily detected (Figures 4-19 and 4-20).

Nicoll and King (1998) evaluated another method of distinguishing tracheal from esophageal intubation. They used a simple adaptation of an ordinary stethoscope inserted into the patient end of the breathing system. Their technique is called *airway auscultation*. Characteristic sounds are heard with the stethoscope during inflation and deflation of the lungs, allowing the observer to diagnose the position of the tube. When the tube is in the trachea (i.e., correctly positioned), loud breath sounds are heard. In contrast, when the tube is in the esophagus (i.e., incorrectly positioned), either squeaks or a flatuslike noise is heard, or no sound at all is heard. In 100 healthy adults, two observers rapidly identified 99 in-

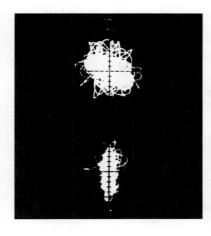

FIGURE 4-20. Lung sound patterns resulting from ventilation of trachea *(upper trace)* and right mainstem bronchus *(lower trace)* in the same patient. (From Huang KC, Kraman SS, Wright BD: *Anesth Analg* 62:586-589, 1983. Reprinted with permission from the International Anesthesia Research Society.)

tubations correctly in a randomized single-blind trial. Nicoll and King recommend further widespread evaluation of airway auscultation because it appears to be an effective, simple, and rapid method of detecting esophageal intubation and confirming tracheal intubation.

Chapter Review and Critical Thinking Questions

1. *Name and describe the four types of breath sounds heard over the normal chest.*

2. *Where are the normal vesicular breath sounds produced? What type of airflow causes these sounds?*

3. *Describe the regional differences in sound intensity at the apex and base of the lung.*

4. *What effect does contraction of the ventricles of the heart have on breath sounds heard over the left lower lobe?*

5. *Why are breath sounds heard at the mouth different from those heard through the chest wall?*

6. *Why do breath sounds heard over the chest fade out during expiration, while those over the trachea do not?*

7. *Does laryngeal noise transmitted to the chest wall form part of the normal vesicular breath sounds?*

BIBLIOGRAPHY

Austrheim O, Kraman SS: The effect of low density gas breathing on vesicular lung sounds, *Respir Physiol* 60:145-155, 1985.

Banaszak EF, Kory RC, Snider GL: Phonopneumography, *Am Rev Respir Dis* 107:449-455, 1973.

Bullar JF: Experiments to determine the origin of the respiratory sounds, *Proc R Soc Lond* 37:411-423, 1884.

Bushnell GE: The mode of production of the so-called vesicular murmur of respiration, *JAMA* 77:2104-2106, 1921.

Cugell DW: Use of tape recordings of respiratory sound and breathing pattern for instruction in pulmonary auscultation, *Am Rev Respir Dis* 104:948-950, 1971.

Dosani R, Kraman SS: Lung sound intensity variability in normal men: a contour phonopneumographic study, *Chest* 83:628-631, 1983.

Forgacs P: *Lung sounds,* London, 1978, Baillière Tindall.

Hannon RR, Lyman RS: Studies on pulmonary acoustics. II. The transmission of tracheal sounds through freshly exenterated sheep's lungs, *Am Rev Tuberc* 19:360-375, 1929.

Hidalgo HA, Wegmann MJ, Waring WW: Frequency spectra of normal breath sounds in childhood, *Chest* 100:999-1002, 1991.

Huang KC, Kraman SS, Wright BD: Video stethoscope: a simple method for assuring continuous bilateral lung ventilation during anesthesia, *Anesth Analg* 62:586-589, 1983.

Kanga JF, Kraman SS: Comparison of the lung sounds frequency spectra of infants and adults, *Pediatr Pulmonol* 2:292-295, 1986.

Kraman SS: Determination of the site of production of respiratory sounds by subtraction phonopneumography, *Am Rev Respir Dis* 122:303-309, 1980.

Kraman SS: Does laryngeal noise contribute to the vesicular lung sound? *Am Rev Respir Dis* 124:292-294, 1981.

Kraman SS: Lung sounds: relative sites of origin and comparative amplitudes in normal subjects, *Lung* 161:57-64, 1983.

Kraman SS: Speed of low-frequency sound through the lungs of normal men, *J Appl Physiol* 55:1862-1867, 1983.

Kraman SS: The relationship between airflow and lung sound amplitude in normal subjects, *Chest* 86:225-229, 1984.

Kraman SS: Effects of lung volume and airflow on the frequency spectrum of vesicular lung sounds, *Respir Physiol* 66:1-9, 1986.

Kraman SS, Austrheim O: Comparison of lung sound and transmitted sound amplitude in normal men, *Clin Res* 31:418A, 1983.

Laennec RTH: *A treatise on the diseases of the chest and mediate auscultation,* New York, 1935, Samuel Wood and Sons (Translated by J Forbes).

Leblanc P, Macklem PT, Ross WRD: Breath sounds and distribution of pulmonary ventilation, *Am Rev Respir Dis* 102:10-16, 1970.

Martini P, Müller H: Studien über das Bronchialatmen, *Dtsch Arch Klin Med* 143:159-173, 1923.

McKusick VA, Jenkins JT, Webb GN: The acoustic basis of the chest examination: studies by means of sound spectrography, *Am Rev Tuberc* 72:12-34, 1955.

Murphy RL: Auscultation of the lung: past lessons, future possibilities, *Thorax* 36:99-107, 1981.

Murphy RL, Holford SK, Knowler WC: Visual lung sound characterization by time expanded waveform analysis, *N Engl J Med* 296:968-971, 1977.

Nairn JR, Turner-Warwick M: Breath sounds in emphysema, *Br J Dis Chest* 63:29-37, 1969.

Nicoll SJ, King CJ: Airway auscultation: a new method of confirming tracheal intubation, *Anaesthesia* 53:41-45, 1998.

O'Donnell DM, Kraman SS: Vesicular lung sound amplitude mapping by automated flow-gated phonopneumography, *J Appl Physiol* 53:603-609, 1982.

Pasterkamp H, Kraman SS, Wodicka GR: Respiratory sounds. Advances beyond the stethoscope, *Am J Respir Crit Care Med* 156:974-987, 1997.

Pasterkamp H, Patel S, Wodicka GR: Asymmetry of respiratory sounds and thoracic transmission, *Med Biol Eng Comput* 35:103-106, 1997.

Ploysongsang Y, Iyer VK, Ramamoorthy PA: Reproducibility of the vesicular breath sounds in normal subjects, *Respiration* 58:158-162, 1991.

Ploysongsang Y, Martin RR, Ross WRD et al: Breath sounds and regional ventilation, *Am Rev Respir Dis* 116:187-199, 1977.

Shykoff BE, Ploysongsang Y, Chang HK: Airflow and normal lung sounds, *Am Rev Respir Dis* 137:872-876, 1988.

Weiss EB, Carlson CJ: Recording of breath sounds, *Am Rev Respir Dis* 105:835-939, 1972.

Chapter 5

Abnormal Breath Sounds

A diseased lung generates many distinctive sounds. These may be roughly grouped into two broad categories: (1) adventitious (accidental) sounds—crackles, wheezes, pleural friction rubs; and (2) abnormally transmitted sounds—egophony, pectoriloquy, bronchophony, bronchial breathing, and abnormally diminished breath sounds. Recent scientific investigations, aided by advances in acoustics and electronics, provide insights into the mechanism of production of these sounds.

TERMINOLOGY: MAKING A CASE FOR CONSISTENCY

When Laennec first described adventitious lung sounds in the nineteenth century, he classified them as "rales" and then added adjectives for further clarification: crepitant (crackling), sibilant (high-pitched), and sonorous (low-pitched). But "rale" had an unpleasant association with the rattle of the secretions in the airways of the dying. To spare the feelings of these patients, Laennec used the synonym "rhonchus" (Greek for *snore*) at the bedside (Robertson and Cope, 1957). Over the years, clinicians added many other adjectives, which, in fact, have no precise meaning and should not be used: wet rales, dry rales, sticky rales, bubbling rales, atelectic rales, and consonating rales (Cugell, 1978; Hudson et al., 1976). To confuse matters still more, "rhonchus" and "wheeze" came to be used interchangeably.

In 1975 the Joint Committee on Pulmonary Nomenclature of the American College of Chest Physicians-American Thoracic Society recategorized the two principal adventitious sounds: (1) "rale" for a discontinuous sound, also called a *crackle;* and (2) "rhonchus" for a continuous sound, which also could be called a *wheeze.*

In 1980 the American Thoracic Society further recategorized these sounds: (1) crackles (coarse and fine), (2) wheeze, and (3) rhonchus.

British investigators using acoustic criteria have modified the terminology for adventitious sounds still further by using only the terms crackle (coarse and fine) and wheeze (high-pitched and low-pitched). The

British terms are used in this chapter. The reader should be aware that in the pulmonary literature, a high-pitched wheeze may be called a *sibilant rhonchus,* whereas a low-pitched wheeze may be referred to as a *sonorous rhonchus.* Moreover, coarse crackles may be called *low-pitched crackles,* and fine crackles may be called *high-pitched crackles.*

ADVENTITIOUS SOUNDS

Crackles

Crackles are short, explosive, nonmusical sounds. In addition to the coarse and fine classification mentioned previously, they may be described as to quantity (scanty or profuse) and timing (inspiratory or expiratory, early or late). They may be heard through the chest wall and sometimes at the mouth.

Laennec gave a very good qualitative description of the crackling sound; he compared it with the sound produced by heating salt in a frying pan. Modern time-expanded waveform analysis shows that the two sounds are indeed quite similar (Murphy, 1981).

In the past, crackles were attributed to bubbling secretions in the airways. This explanation is probably correct when the trachea and main bronchi are full of sputum and when the crackling is both inspiratory and expiratory. However, in other diseases in which there is no sputum, and when crackling is confined to inspiration, this explanation cannot be valid (Forgacs, 1978b).

The most widely accepted cause of crackling, described by Dr. Paul Forgacs, is the explosive equalization of gas pressure between two compartments of the lung, when a closed section of the airways separating them suddenly opens (Figure 5-1). Several observations lend support to this notion.

In excised lungs, inflation is not accompanied by crackling unless the lung is deflated at the start of the experiment to the point at which some groups of alveoli under the pleura are seen to be airless. Under these circumstances, the lung does not inflate smoothly or evenly; instead, small groups of alveoli expand suddenly all over the surface. This random reinflation is accompanied by crackling, which stops as soon as the whole lung is reaerated.

Another important clue to the genesis of crackling is the recurrent rhythm, characterized by similar spacing and relative loudness of successive crackles, that can often be recognized in several consecutive respiratory cycles (Figure 5-2). The recurrent rhythm indicates that the airways responsible for individual crackles open in the same sequence and at approximately the same lung volume. Nath and Capel (1974b) have confirmed that the reopening of each airway and, therefore, the timing of each crackle are closely linked to the transpulmonary pressure; this was accomplished by simultaneous recording of sound amplitude and

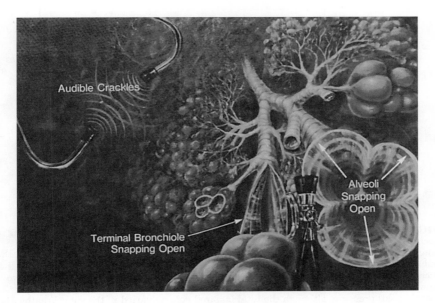

FIGURE 5-1. The primary source of crackling is the explosive equalization of gas pressure between two compartments of the lung when a closed section of airway separating them suddenly opens. (Illustration by Edward M. Jones.)

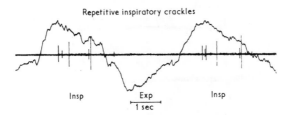

FIGURE 5-2. Simultaneous recording of inspiratory crackles and airflow rate shows a repetitive pattern of crackles *(short vertical lines)* in the two breaths. (From Nath AR, Capel LH: *Thorax* 29:695-698, 1974. Reprinted by permission of the *New England Journal of Medicine.*)

esophageal pressure, which is equivalent to pleural pressure. In several consecutive respiratory cycles, crackles, identified by their spacing and relative amplitude, occurred at the same transpulmonary pressure (Figure 5-3). The significance of these experiments is that these crackles, because of their close relationship to transpulmonary pressure and their similarity in each respiratory cycle, must be the result of the sudden opening of airways. They cannot be caused by bubbling secretions in the airways; if they were, they would not be related to transpulmonary pressure and would not sound similar in each respiratory cycle.

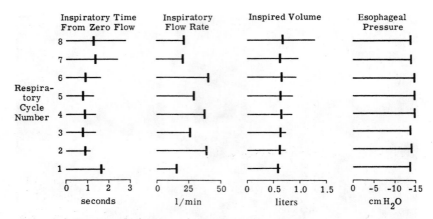

FIGURE 5-3. Results of experiment showing that reopening of each airway and timing of each crackle are closely linked to the transpulmonary pressure. From left to right, the length of the horizontal line represents the inspiratory time, the inspiratory flow rate, the inspired volume, and the transpulmonary pressure. The short vertical line represents the occurrence of a particular crackle, repeating through eight breaths. Note in the last two columns that the crackle occurred at a similar inspired volume and transpulmonary (esophageal) pressure, although the total inspired volume varied in the eight breaths. But the occurrence of this crackle is not closely related to the inspiratory time and inspiratory flow rate (*first two columns*). (From Nath AR, Capel LH: *Thorax* 29:695-698, 1974. Reprinted by permission of the *New England Journal of Medicine.*)

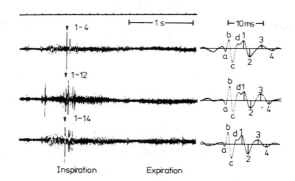

FIGURE 5-4. Amplitude versus time plots of lung sounds recorded from a patient with pulmonary tuberculosis and thoracoplasty during three consecutive respiratory cycles. Note the repetitive appearance of crackles with almost identical waveforms. The *starting segment* of the waveform *(abcd)* and the *decay segment (1234)* can also be seen. (From Mori M, Kinoshita M, Morinari H et al: *Thorax* 35:843-850, 1980. Reprinted by permission of the *New England Journal of Medicine.*)

In Japan, Mori and colleagues (1980) have used the technique of time-expanded waveform analysis to study crackles, elaborating on the work of Nath and Capel. Mori and associates found that crackles occurred at the same point in the respiratory cycle and that repetitive crackles had identical waveforms (Figure 5-4). Characteristically, the

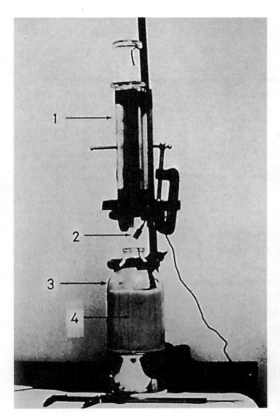

FIGURE 5-5. Crackle simulator consisting of a syringe *(1)*, a microphone *(2)*, and a bottle *(3)*, with its internal surface covered with polyurethane foam *(4)*. The simulated crackles are produced by applying commercial paste to the orifice of the syringe and moving the piston up and down slowly. The vernier caliper at the bottom indicates 5 cm. The waveforms generated are similar to those of actual crackles. (From Mori M, Kinoshita K, Morinari H et al: *Thorax* 35:843-850, 1980. Reprinted by permission of the *New England Journal of Medicine.*)

waveforms were separable into two segments, an initial "starting segment" and a subsequent "decay segment." The starting segment is apparently a shock wave caused by the abrupt opening of an airway. The subsequent decay segment is the result of the shock wave exciting a resonator in the lung. To test this shock wave-resonator hypothesis, they constructed a crackle simulator consisting of a syringe, a microphone, and a bottle resonator (Figure 5-5) and successfully obtained waveforms similar to those of crackles.

Nath and Capel (1974a, 1980) have shown that the timing of crackles in the inspiratory cycle can be used to distinguish the pulmonary diseases, which are discussed next.

Crackles in Obstructive Disease
Early inspiratory crackles (Figure 5-6) are characteristic of patients with severe airway obstruction. These crackles appear to be produced in the proximal and larger airways. They are frequently well transmitted to the mouth, are few in number, and are heard at one or both lung bases. An

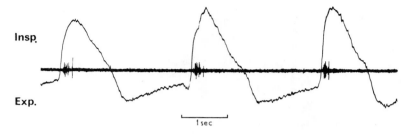

FIGURE 5-6. Phonopneumogram of early inspiratory crackles *(short vertical lines)*. Note that this is a simultaneous recording of both the crackles and the airflow rate. (From Nath AR, Capel LH: *Thorax* 29:223-227, 1974. Reprinted by permission of the *New England Journal of Medicine.*)

important feature of these crackles is that they are not silenced by cough or change of posture. Some of the diseases they appear in are discussed in the following sections.

Chronic Bronchitis. Chronic bronchitis produces excessive secretion of mucus, resulting in chronic cough productive of sputum. Pathologically, bronchitis is characterized by proliferation and hyperplasia of the mucous glands in the large airways, extending abnormally into small airways, often without evidence of inflammatory changes, although the changes may be associated with bacterial infection. Chronic bronchitis is commonly caused by the inhalation of cigarette smoke, although the disease is found in a few nonsmokers as well, particularly miners and persons living in polluted urban environments. The principal complication associated with chronic bronchitis is the development of obstructive airway disease.

Asthma. Asthma is the result of reversible airway obstruction and hyperirritability of the airways. Substances that have no effect when inhaled by normal persons cause bronchoconstriction in asthmatics. The severity of asthma is extremely variable, ranging from mild symptoms in children, which may disappear in later life, to severe, continuous, and even fatal obstruction of the airways. Although asthma does not cause emphysema or other chronic diseases, it may itself be a significant cause of disability.

Emphysema. Emphysema is an abnormal enlargement of the air spaces accompanied by destruction of the alveolar walls, resulting in considerable increase in the volume of the lungs (described more fully in Chapter 1).

Crackles in Restrictive Disease

Late inspiratory crackles are characteristic of patients with restrictive pulmonary disease (Figure 5-7). They are usually more numerous than early inspiratory crackles, vary with patient position, and are only rarely

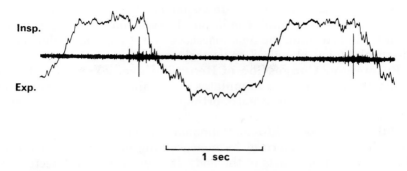

FIGURE 5-7. Phonopneumogram of inspiratory crackles occurring late in inspiration. (From Nath AR, Capel LH: *Thorax* 29:223-227, 1974. Reprinted by permission of the *New England Journal of Medicine.*)

transmitted to the mouth. They appear to originate in peripheral airways, each crackle representing the abrupt opening of a single airway. Occasionally, late inspiratory crackles are associated with a short end-inspiratory wheeze. These crackles are seen in the following diseases.

Interstitial Fibrosis. Interstitial fibrosis, also called *interstitial pneumonitis,* is associated with interstitial and alveolar infiltrates and fibrosis. Patients complain of cough; of difficulty in breathing; and, rarely, of fever. Pulmonary function studies show restriction and are sensitive indicators of the extent of the illness. Interstitial fibrosis may be caused by cancer chemotherapeutic agents (bleomycin, cyclophosphamide, methotrexate), radiation therapy, the antibiotic nitrofurantoin, high oxygen concentrations inhaled over a long period, and heavy metals such as gold; it is most often idiopathic.

Asbestosis. Asbestos is widely used in many industries; shipworkers, insulators, and persons who work with brake linings and asbestos shingles are vulnerable to asbestosis. Inhalation of the tiny asbestos particles leads to pulmonary inflammation and fibrosis. Another disease associated with asbestos exposure, lung cancer, develops particularly among cigarette smokers. Persons exposed to asbestos also have increased incidence of cancer of the abdominal organs and mesothelioma. Asbestos particles, found in the lungs of nearly all city dwellers, are an extremely potent disease-causing agent; persons who have merely worked in shipyards, even if not directly exposed to asbestos, often have asbestos bodies in their lungs and are at high risk to contract lung cancer. In addition, the families of asbestos workers and people living near plants using asbestos have increased risk of lung cancer, which may not occur until 20 or 30 years after exposure.

Pneumonia. An inflammation of the lungs, pneumonia continues to be a major health problem in the United States and, despite antibiotic treatment, an important cause of death. It ranges in severity from a mild illness with a small lung infiltrate visible on chest radiograph to an extensive, progressive, fatal condition. Pneumonia is most commonly caused by a bacterium, the pneumococcus, but it may be nonbacterial as well—viral, fungal, chemical, or mycoplasmal.

Pulmonary Congestion of Heart Failure. When the left ventricle fails, the lung tissue accumulates excess fluid. Patients complain of progressive shortness of breath, orthopnea, and paroxysmal nocturnal dyspnea.

Pulmonary Sarcoidosis. Pulmonary sarcoidosis is a chronic, often benign disease characterized by noncaseating granulomas in the lung and frequently other parts of the body. It is usually first detected as bilaterally enlarged asymptomatic lymph nodes in the lung hila. The cause is unknown but is believed to be ingestion of a specific substance that provokes an immune reaction. In less than one third of cases, the lung eventually becomes scarred with interstitial fibrosis, leading to restricted pulmonary function.

Scleroderma. Scleroderma, more properly called *systemic sclerosis* or *generalized scleroderma,* is a disease of connective tissue and is manifested by dermal fibrosis, atrophy of the skin, and fixation of the skin to underlying structures. Systemically, patients develop muscle wasting, joint deformity, diminished esophageal and small bowel function, respiratory insufficiency with pulmonary fibrosis and restriction of lung function, and scleroderma of the kidney followed by renal failure. Scleroderma also frequently affects the heart. The disease affects women three times as frequently as men, with onset usually between the ages of 20 and 55. The cause is unknown.

Rheumatoid Lung. Rheumatoid arthritis is a systemic disease that causes inflammatory changes in connective tissue throughout the body and commonly damages the smaller joints—proximal interphalangeal, metacarpophalangeal, and metatarsophalangeal. Three times as many women as men are affected, with the average age of onset being 35 years. In the lung, the disease causes diffuse interstitial fibrosis, pleural effusions, and nodular lesions. The cause of rheumatoid arthritis is unknown.

Fine and Coarse Crackles

Fine and coarse crackles occur in different lung diseases. Fine crackles are commonly associated with pulmonary fibrosis. Coarse crackles are a characteristic finding in bronchiectasis (discussed in the following section). Time-expanded waveform analysis (Figure 5-8) demonstrates that the early and late segments of fine and coarse crackles have different characteristics, probably related to the origin of the sound and the resonance of the lung (Munakata et al., 1991).* Jones and colleagues (2000)

---

* Bettencourt and others (1994) have used time-expanded waveform analysis to diagnose common pulmonary conditions and report that the method performs well.

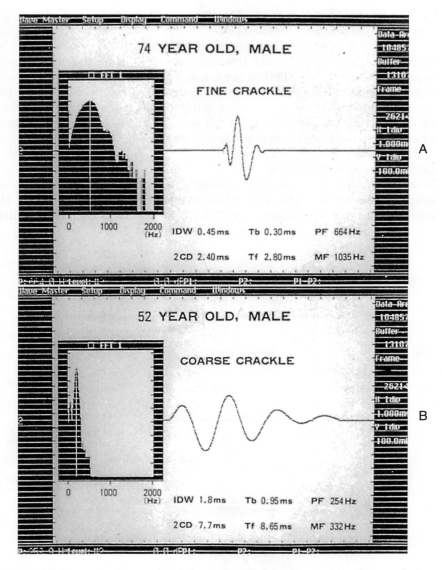

FIGURE 5-8. Example of time-expanded waveform and fast Fourier transform analysis of fine **(A)** and coarse **(B)** crackles. *2CD,* The duration of the first two cycles of the crackle waveform; *IDW,* initial deflection width, the duration of the first-half cycle of the crackle waveform; *MF,* maximum frequency; *PF,* peak frequency; *Tb,* the duration of the first-quarter cycle of the crackle waveform; *Tf,* the duration of the first 9/4 cycles of the crackle waveform. (From Munakata M, Ukita H, Doi I et al: *Thorax* 46:651-657, 1991.)

have suggested that coarse crackles may result from the explosion of gas bubbles in pulmonary secretions.

Figure 5-8 also demonstrates the analysis of fine and coarse crackles by computerized fast Fourier transformation. This mathematical technique transforms a segment of the crackle sound into a spectrum of constituent sound intensities and displays them in relation to sound frequency. Fast Fourier transformation is the most important new procedure for quantifying and analyzing breath sounds. It has been used to study wheezes, transmitted voice sounds, and crackles (*Lancet*, 1986).

Crackles in Bronchiectasis

Bronchiectasis is a permanent dilation of the airways that may be very similar to bronchitis. The form of airway enlargement ranges from the generalized cylindric dilation of chronic bronchitis to saccular outpouch-

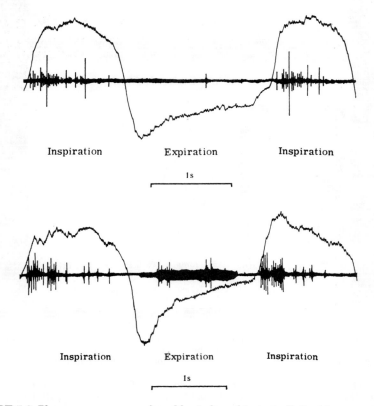

FIGURE 5-9. Phonopneumograms of crackles in bronchiectasis. Patient in upper tracing had chronic bronchitis and bronchiectasis; tracing shows early and midinspiratory crackles. Patient in lower tracing had bronchiectasis and lung fibrosis; paninspiratory and expiratory crackles are seen. Lung crackles here are more profuse in early and midinspiration. (From Nath AR, Capel LH: *Thorax* 35:694-699, 1980.)

ings from more localized disease. Bronchiectasis has many causes: airway obstruction by a tumor or foreign body, viral and bacterial pneumonia, tuberculosis, chronic inflammatory or fibrotic pulmonary disease, and heroin-induced pulmonary edema. The crackles of bronchiectasis typically occur in early and midphase inspiration, and airway obstruction is mild (Figure 5-9); they are coarse and more profuse than most other early inspiratory crackles, independent of patient position, usually present in expiration, and become less numerous after coughing. In Table 5-1, the crackles of bronchiectasis are compared with those of other lung diseases.

Crackles are not necessarily an abnormal finding. For example, Thacker and Kraman (1982) were able to record crackles anteriorly in 26 of 52 normal subjects (mostly male) when they inhaled deeply from residual volume. These crackles were commonly profuse and loud. Waveform analysis showed them to be like the crackles of interstitial lung disease. Workum and associates (1982) have obtained similar results in normal women. Both groups found these crackles to be rarely, if ever, heard during breathing from resting lung volume.

The incidence of crackles is important in the diagnosis of pulmonary disease. For example, Epler and colleagues (1978) have reported that bilateral high-pitched crackles are heard in 60% of patients with interstitial pneumonias and asbestosis but in only 20% of those with sarcoidosis and other granulomatoses (Figures 5-10 and 5-11). In asbestosis, high-pitched crackles correlated with pathologic severity, with honeycombing changes in the lung on radiograph, and with physiologic abnormalities. Furthermore, the presence of bilateral basal crackles is closely related to the duration of asbestos exposure; these crackles often occur before asbestosis is detected on chest radiograph (Shirai et al., 1981) (Figure 5-12). Therefore, although crackles are not always abnormal, they should be listened for in a patient with a history suggestive of disease. Al Jared and

TABLE 5-1. Crackles in Various Lung Diseases*

Condition	Associated Crackles
Healthy	Fine crackles at anterior bases, only during inspiration from low lung volume
Idiopathic interstitial fibrosis	Prominent fine crackles
Asbestosis	Prominent fine crackles, may be first indication of disease
Bronchiectasis	Coarse crackles, often heard at the mouth
Chronic bronchitis	Coarse crackles, often heard at the mouth
Congestive heart failure	Fine crackles
Sarcoidosis	Sparse fine crackles
Miliary tuberculosis	Sparse fine crackles
Other granulomatous lung diseases	Sparse fine crackles

From Kraman SS: *Arch Intern Med* 146:1411-1412, 1986. Copyright 1986, American Medical Association.
*For a description of identifiable characteristics of fine and coarse crackles, see text.

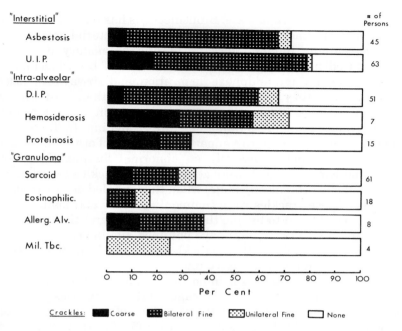

FIGURE 5-10. Types of crackles according to pathologic diagnosis in 272 patients with chronic infiltrative pulmonary disease diagnosed by biopsy. *Allerg. Alv.,* Allergic alveolitis; *D.I.P.,* desquamative interstitial pneumonia; *Mil. Tbc.,* miliary tuberculosis; *U.I.P.,* unusual interstitial pneumonia. (From Epler GR, Carrington CB, Gaensler EA: *Chest* 73:333-339, 1978.)

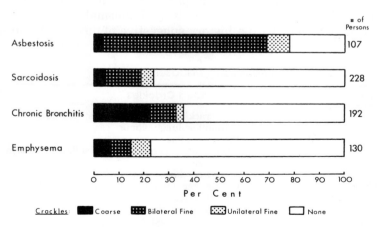

FIGURE 5-11. Incidence and types of crackles according to clinical diagnoses in 657 patients. Note that crackles were most common in asbestosis. (From Epler GR, Carrington CB, Gaensler EA: *Chest* 73:333-339, 1978.)

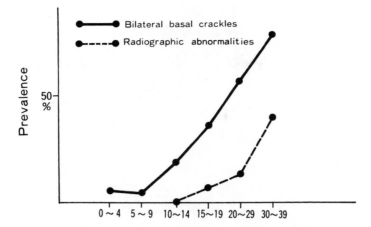

FIGURE 5-12. Bilateral basal crackles and radiographic abnormalities in asbestos workers—relationship between prevalence and duration of exposure. Note that crackles occurred before radiographic abnormalities. (From Shirai F, Kudoh S, Shibuya A et al: *Br J Dis Chest* 75:386-396, 1981.)

associates (1993) report that time-expanded waveform analysis is even more sensitive than auscultation in detecting inspiratory crackles in asbestos workers.

Crackles also should be searched for in patients who have just suffered a myocardial infarction. Crackles that appear over the upper two thirds of the posterior lung fields, while the patient is still in the coronary care unit, are an extremely bad sign. A patient with such crackles is 3.3 times more likely to die in the 2-year period following the infarct than is the same patient without these crackles. Crackles heard only at the lung bases—that is the lower third of the posterior lung fields—do not have the same dire significance.

The exact cardiac abnormality that causes the crackles over the upper two thirds of the posterior lung fields is as yet uncertain. Surprisingly, they are unrelated to radionuclide ejection fraction, a technique used to assess the function of the left ventricle (Multicenter Postinfarction Research Group, 1983).

In myocardial infarct patients without obvious congestive heart failure, Deguchi and others (1993) found that fine crackles could be induced by changing posture from sitting to supine and/or from supine to supine with passive leg elevation (Figure 5-13). They named these fine crackles *posturally induced crackles*. To investigate the relationship between posturally induced crackles and long-term prognosis after myocardial infarction, Deguchi and associates followed up 262 patients who recovered from acute myocardial infarction for a mean period of 6 years. Using a

Sitting

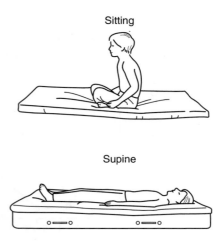

Supine

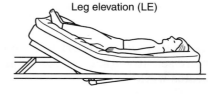

Leg elevation (LE)

FIGURE 5-13. Positions for examining a subject to identify posturally induced crackles. (From Deguchi F, Hirakawa S, Gotoh K: *Chest* 103:1457-1462, 1993.)

multilogistic model, they found that posturally induced crackles were the third most important prognostic factor, after number of diseased coronary vessels and pulmonary capillary wedge pressure.

Figure 5-14 summarizes the incidence and characteristics of crackles in asbestosis, left ventricular heart failure, and asbestos-related pleural disease.

Wheezes

A wheeze (rhonchus) is a musical pulmonary sound. The musical character, obvious to any listener, is determined by the spectrum of frequencies that make up the sound. The lowest or fundamental frequency sets the pitch of the note.

The musical character of the wheezing sound can be recognized on a phonopneumogram by the regular pattern formed by a sequence of identical waveforms (Figure 5-15). Wheezes are classified as high- or low-pitched, inspiratory or expiratory, short or long, and single or multiple. A monophonic wheeze consists of a single note or of several notes starting and ending at different times. A polyphonic wheeze is made up of several dissonant notes starting and ending simultaneously, like a chord.

Percentage of Inspiratory
crackles

Timing of crackles during the respiratory cycle

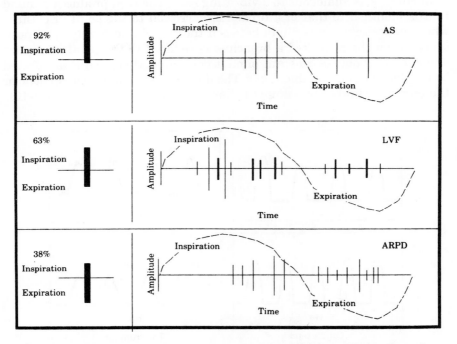

FIGURE 5-14. Summary of the incidence and characteristics of crackles in asbestosis *(AS)*, left ventricular failure *(LVF)*, and asbestos-related pleural disease *(ARPD)*. (From al Jarad N, Davies SW, Logan-Sinclair R et al: *Respir Med* 88:37-46, 1994.)

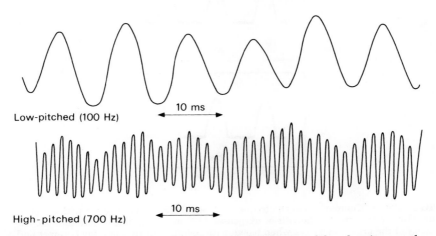

FIGURE 5-15. Waveforms of a wheeze. The musical character of the wheezing sound can be recognized by the regular pattern formed by a sequence of identical waveforms. (From Forgacs P: *Lung sounds,* London, 1978, Baillière Tindall.)

The most widely accepted mechanism of wheezing, described by Dr. Paul Forgacs, is analogous to a vibrating reed. The reed produces a sound that is identical to that of a bronchus narrowed to the point of closure, whose opposite walls oscillate between the closed and barely open positions. When the caliber of a bronchus is reduced to the point of closure and a musical note of constant pitch is generated, this pitch is unaffected by the density of the ambient gas. The detached mouthpiece of an oboe or the reed of a child's toy trumpet behaves in the same way (Figure 5-16).

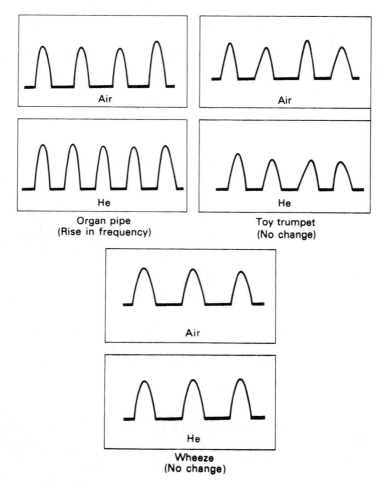

FIGURE 5-16. Comparison of the frequency of wind instruments blown with air or helium (He) and a wheeze when air or oxygen and helium are inhaled. Note that the frequency of the organ pipe rises when blown with helium, but that of a toy trumpet and a wheeze do not change. This indicates that a wheeze is produced by a vibrating reed-type mechanism that, like the vibrating reed in the toy trumpet, is unaffected by the density of the ambient gas. (From Forgacs P: *Lung sounds,* London, 1978, Baillière Tindall.)

The vibrating reed mechanism makes it incorrect to attribute high-pitched wheezing to short peripheral airways and low-pitched wheezing to long central bronchi. It is true that the oscillations of a large mass, such as a tumor occluding a main bronchus, usually produce a low-pitched note. Nevertheless, high-pitched wheezing may be generated centrally or peripherally and may rise or fall during a single respiratory cycle in parallel with the tightness of the compression.

For many years, investigators believed that the musical sound of wheezing was generated in a manner similar to sound production within an organ pipe. The gas within a narrowed bronchus was supposed to be set into oscillation in much the same way as a stream of air blown across a flue pipe, producing a musical note whose pitch was determined by the dimensions of the pipe. Thus a simple reduction in the pipe caliber or a spur facing the stream of gas in the airway was assumed sufficient to generate musical sounds; the pitch of the note would depend on the length of the adjoining airway. High-pitched wheezing was therefore often attributed to peripheral bronchial spasm.

Although this theory of wheezing may be attractive, it is contradicted by several facts: (1) The longest axial pathway in the bronchial tree is less than 1 foot, whereas the frequency of some low-pitched wheezes is in the range produced by pipes 4 to 8 feet long. (2) Unlike the sound of an organ pipe, the pitch of a wheeze emanating from a stenosed bronchus is not fixed; indeed, it may differ by as much as an octave between inspiration and expiration. In experiments with excised bronchi, no musical sound results from a simple reduction in caliber until the opposite walls of the compressed bronchus are brought into contact. The frequency of the note can then be varied over several octaves by tightening the compression or increasing the blowing pressure. (3) The definitive argument against the organ pipe model is that the pitch of the tone rises when the pipe is blown with helium, a less dense gas than air. However, the pitch of a wheeze stays constant when the inspired air is replaced by a mixture of helium and oxygen (Forgacs, 1978b).

Monophonic Wheezes

A characteristic example of a monophonic wheeze is the single musical tone made by a bronchus that is almost completely occluded by tumor. If the narrowing is rigid, the wheeze can be heard throughout the respiratory cycle; if the narrowing is flexible, the wheeze may not be audible during either inspiration or expiration, especially if the patient is turned from one side to the other. Single or multiple monophonic wheezes are a characteristic clinical sign of asthma. The number of wheezes is never large; the illusion that many wheezes are heard under the stethoscope results from the wide transmission of a few loud wheezes with varying relative intensity to different points on the chest wall.

In asbestosis and interstitial fibrosis, an unusual type of monophonic wheezing is occasionally heard over the lower regions of the lung. It is restricted to inspiration and is often associated with late inspiratory crackling. Some of these patients have a single short wheeze at the end of inspiration; others have several short wheezes of different pitch following one another throughout inspiration.

As was mentioned, late inspiratory crackles and an end-inspiratory wheeze are often associated. That both are heard over deflated regions of the lung suggests that their mode of production is similar. Apparently, end-inspiratory wheezes are produced by airways whose walls oscillate in apposition for a few milliseconds before opening fully. Because these airways open at a predetermined transpulmonary pressure, the same sequence of musical notes will occur in several consecutive respiratory cycles (Forgacs, 1978b).

Polyphonic Wheezes

Polyphonic wheezing is a frequent sign of most types of chronic obstructive pulmonary disease. It is confined largely to expiration and, as was mentioned, comprises several dissonant notes starting and ending at the same time.

A polyphonic wheeze is produced by compression of the central bronchi. Although it is a reliable sign of widespread obstruction to airflow, polyphonic wheezing also can be generated in normal subjects, in whom it is called a *forced expiratory wheeze* (Kraman, 1983). There are two ways to differentiate a forced expiratory wheeze from a pathologic polyphonic wheeze:

1. A forced expiratory wheeze can be produced in normal subjects only during a violent expiratory effort. In contrast, patients with severe airflow obstruction will wheeze even during a gentle expiration.
2. In a healthy subject, during a forced expiration, the progressively louder breath sounds will retain their character as *white noise* until a strong expiratory effort, delivered with maximum force, suddenly evokes the full complement of musical sounds contained in the forced expiratory wheeze. (As noted in Chapter 4, white noise is made up of sound waves of many different frequencies and is analogous to white light, which comprises light waves of many different frequencies.) In contrast, subjects with diseased lungs produce a sequence of musical sounds, starting with a monophonic wheeze at a mildly forced expiration and progressing to bitonal and multiple wheezes with increased effort; the full polyphonic wheeze eventually follows (Forgacs, 1978b).

Polyphonic wheezing is heard in all forms of obstructive lung disease, asthma and emphysema being examples. An abnormal polyphonic wheeze is the direct result of pathologic changes that have taken place within the bronchi. In contrast, the forced expiratory wheeze does not result from pathologic changes—simply from a high rate of airflow.

Stridor and Hoarseness

Stridor is a particularly loud musical sound of constant pitch, most prominent during inspiration, and heard very well at a distance from the patient. Although nothing except its intensity distinguishes stridor from a monophonic wheeze, which cannot be heard at a distance from the patient, the term is widely used when laryngeal or tracheal obstruction is known or suspected to be the source of the sound (Forgacs, 1978b).

The mechanism of stridor, like that of wheezing, is analogous to a vibrating reed. The reed produces a sound that is identical to a larynx or trachea narrowed to the point of closure, whose opposite walls oscillate between the closed and barely open positions; they all produce a musical note of constant pitch. However, stridor is generated in central airways, whereas wheezing comes from more peripheral airways.

Although stridor is typically inspiratory, it becomes inspiratory and expiratory as the airway becomes increasingly obstructed, as by laryngeal tumors, tracheal stenosis, or an aspirated foreign body. When particularly severe, stridor is associated with gasping respiration and use of the accessory muscles of respiration.

Hoarseness is a roughened, coarse quality of the voice, occurring whenever a normal, smooth vocal cord is not brought into contact with its fellow. Hoarseness indicates either that there are irregularities on the surface of one or both cords or that there is a disorder of nerves and muscles responsible for vocal cord movement. Hoarseness is dealt with in this section because, although not a wheeze, it can be produced by the same pathologic changes in the larynx that cause stridor.

The significance of hoarseness and stridor is different in children and adults. The diseases causing these conditions are discussed in the following section.

Stridor in Children

In a child, obstruction of the airway and trachea is usually much more rapid and life threatening than in an adult. Severe obstruction is accompanied by cyanosis and pallor of the skin, dilation of the nostrils, downward plunging of the trachea, and use of the accessory muscles of respiration. Voice changes, swallowing difficulties, respiratory infections, and failure to thrive are seen in less severe obstruction (Ludman, 1981). There are several causes of airway obstruction in a child.

Laryngomalacia (congenital stridor) is manifested in the first few months of life. Characteristically, the infant appears to be normal except for the stridor, which is particularly audible when the infant is supine or

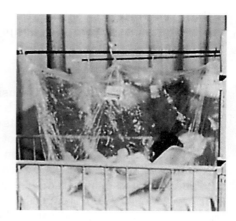

FIGURE 5-17. A hospital croup tent used to treat children with viral croup. (From Valman HB: *BMJ* 283:294-295, 1981.)

excited. Laryngomalacia means softening of the larynx. This, in fact, is what one sees through the laryngoscope. The epiglottis, arytenoid cartilage, and aryepiglottic folds are "floppy" and drawn into the larynx during inspiration. The condition commonly becomes more severe during the first year of life but then gradually improves, with complete recovery.

Viral croup is the most common cause of upper airway obstruction in infants. Most cases occur between October and April in children 3 months to 3 years of age, and boys outnumber girls 2:1. The signs and symptoms usually begin suddenly at night, after several days of upper respiratory infection. The child has stridor and a characteristic barking, croupy cough; anxiety worsens the problem. Tracheostomy or intubation is performed in severe cases; the mortality rate may be as high as 2.7%. Humidity administered by vaporizer, racemic epinephrine by aerosol, steam inhalation at home, and "croup tent" in the hospital (Figure 5-17) are the most common forms of treatment (Roberts, 1979). But the value of steam inhalation can be questioned, especially that administered at home.

Acute epiglottitis (Figure 5-18) is a severe, often fatal infection caused by *Hemophilus influenzae* type B bacteria. The illness develops very rapidly. After a few hours of sore throat and fever, the child's jaw protrudes; he drools, refuses to swallow, and appears anxious. The stridor and other signs result from swelling of the epiglottis and upper portion of the larynx. It is important to recognize this problem and to avoid tongue blade and examination of the throat. Incidence of acute epiglottitis is lower since HIB vaccination. Mortality can be reduced from 24% to 2% by provision of an airway through nasotracheal intubation or tracheostomy. At present, chloramphenicol is the antibiotic of choice. Epiglottitis is ordinarily a brief illness; most patients need the airway for a day or two at most.

Diphtheria, caused by *Corynebacterium diphtheriae,* is quite rare today because of immunization. Nevertheless, it should be suspected if a

RADIOGRAPHIC APPEARANCES

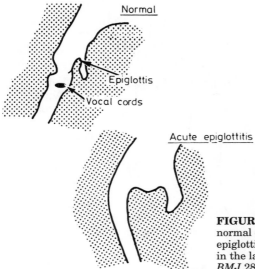

FIGURE 5-18. Appearance of the larynx in normal children and in those with acute epiglottitis. Note the swelling of the epiglottis in the latter condition. (From Valman HB: *BMJ* 283:294-295, 1981.)

dirty gray, tough, fibrinous pseudomembrane is present in the throat in the region of the tonsils. As the disease progresses, swelling of the pharynx and larynx obstructs breathing. When untreated, death may result from complete, sudden airway obstruction or from heart failure, the result of a toxin produced by the bacteria. Diphtheria antitoxin and antibiotics—procaine penicillin, ampicillin, erythromycin, clindamycin, or rifampin—are an effective form of therapy (Beers and Berkow, 1999). With immunization, the diphtheria epidemics of past centuries have all but disappeared. Medical historians speculate that one such epidemic caused the death of George Washington in 1799.

Laryngeal paralysis at birth is believed to result from the stretching of the vagus nerve during a difficult delivery. The condition is associated with feeding difficulties. The child may prefer to lie with the head turned to one side, and there may be unilateral facial weakness. Spontaneous recovery usually occurs during the first year of life.

Congenital narrowing of the larynx or trachea may be caused by webs between the cords or by narrowing of the space beneath (Figure 5-19). Surgical correction is often necessary.

Inhalation of a foreign body causes 3000 Americans to choke to death annually. Foreign body obstruction of the adult airway occurs commonly while the victim is eating. In a child, choking may occur during play, when a small toy or object being mouthed slips back into the airway. There are four signs of choking: (1) inability to speak or breathe, (2) pallor followed by increasing cyanosis, (3) loss of consciousness and collapse, and (4) the

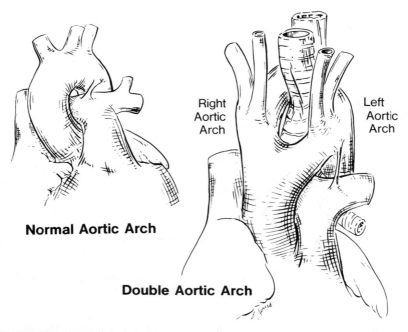

Right
Aortic
Arch

Left
Aortic
Arch

Normal Aortic Arch

Double Aortic Arch

FIGURE 5-19. Congenital narrowing of the trachea caused by a double aortic arch.

so-called Heimlich sign, in which the victim brings his hand to his throat with the thumb and index finger spread wide to form a "V." The foreign body may be dislodged by the Heimlich maneuver (Figure 5-20).

Stridor and Hoarseness in Adults

In an adult, abnormalities of the larynx cause hoarseness more often than they cause stridor. Acute hoarseness, a change in the voice of less than 3 weeks' duration, may be caused by infectious laryngitis; trauma from shouting, coughing, or vomiting; inhalation of smoke or noxious fumes; or allergic swelling (angioedema). Chronic hoarseness—hoarseness of more than 3 weeks' duration—may be the result of the following conditions:

1. *Chronic laryngitis,* a continuing irritation of the laryngeal mucosa, is often a result of straining the voice during an acute attack of laryngitis, with submucosal hemorrhage and vocal cord edema. Tuberculosis and syphilis are uncommon causes. Vocal cord nodules (singer's nodules) develop after chronic voice abuse such as screaming or shouting. They are tiny fibrous nodules of both vocal cords and may be removed surgically.
2. *Vocal cord paralysis* is frequently caused by damage to the recurrent laryngeal nerve. The damage is often inflicted by a can-

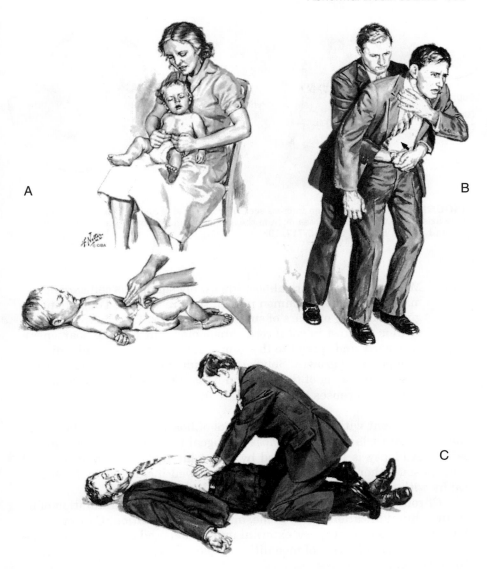

A

B

C

FIGURE 5-20. The Heimlich maneuver. **A,** An infant victim. **B,** Victim standing. **C,** Victim supine. (Copyright 1979, CIBA Pharmaceutical Company, Division of CIBA GEIGY Corporation. Reprinted with permission from CLINICAL SYMPOSIA, illustrated by Frank H. Netter, MD. All rights reserved.)

cer in the hilum of the lung. Sometimes the nerve is injured during thyroidectomy or is affected by neuritis. In many cases no cause is found.

3. *Neoplasms of the larynx* may arise from the vocal cords (glottic) or from above or below them (supraglottic, subglottic) (Figure 5-21).

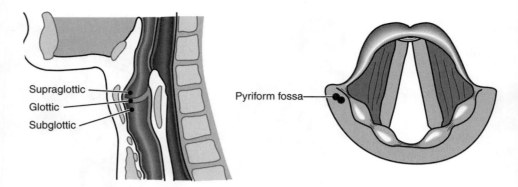

FIGURE 5-21. The larynx seen in cross-section from the side and from above. Tumors may arise from the pyriform fossa or from the subglottic, glottic, or supraglottic regions. (From Ludman H: *BMJ* 282:715-717, 1981.)

Malignant tumors are almost invariably squamous cell carcinomas and are more common in men than in women. The patient gives a history of years of smoking cigarettes. The chance of survival is greatest in vocal cord carcinomas, which cause hoarseness very early and spread to the lymph nodes in the neck only after a long period of growth. Subglottic carcinomas have the worst prognosis. Carcinoma of the pyriform fossa invades the muscles of the larynx and causes hoarseness late in the disease.

Any patient with more than 3 weeks of hoarseness should be examined by indirect laryngoscopy. Most laryngeal tumors can be seen with a mirror. A biopsy is then obtained by direct laryngoscopy under general anesthesia. Other diagnostic methods employed include x-ray laryngography with contrast medium and laryngeal tomography.

Chronic laryngitis is treated by resting of the voice, elimination of irritants, humidification of the home, and steam inhalation. Cancer of the larynx is treated by surgery, external irradiation, and chemotherapy; the modality or combination of modalities employed depends on the extent of the disease.

In an adult, airway obstruction may be caused by large tumors, bilateral paralysis of laryngeal nerves, or inhalation of foreign bodies, particularly lumps of food. The physician can quickly relieve laryngeal obstruction by making an incision over the cricothyroid membrane and inserting a tube. Because the cricothyroid membrane is just below the skin surface, this procedure, called *laryngotomy* (Figure 5-22), is much more simply and safely performed than is tracheostomy. The treatment of choice for inhaled food is the Heimlich maneuver (see Figure 5-20).

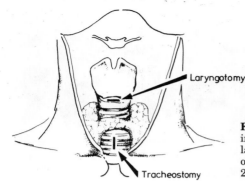

FIGURE 5-22. Diagram of the neck, showing where incisions for tracheostomy and laryngotomy are made to relieve airway obstruction. (From Ludman H: *BMJ* 282:715-717, 1981.)

Sometimes an adult may experience airway obstruction that lacks an identifiable organic cause. Such patients have dramatic episodes of stridor, which may have been mistaken for asthma and ordinary wheezing. The stridor results from complete adduction of the true vocal cords, reducing the glottic opening to a small posterior diamond-shaped chink. Persons with this condition show a variety of psychiatric disorders, ranging from mild stress-related worsening of symptoms to obsessive-compulsive neurosis; they have difficulty in directly expressing anger, sadness, or fear and have various degrees of secondary gain from their respiratory symptoms. Treatment consists of teaching the patients to concentrate on active expiration by using their ventral abdominal muscles and to relax the oropharyngeal muscles. In combination with short-term psychotherapy, these measures immediately reduce both the number and severity of attacks in all patients (Christopher, 1983).

Pleural Friction Rub

The smooth, moist layers of the normal pleura move easily and silently over one another. However, when the surface is coarsened by fibrin deposits or thickened by inflammatory or neoplastic cells, the sliding motion is impeded by frictional resistance. The sound produced resembles that of a stringed instrument. If a large area of the chest wall is involved, the sound is musical.

More commonly, however, the irregular sliding movement of the lung generates a series of nonmusical sounds, usually longer and of lower pitch than lung crackles; a characteristic pleural friction rub has been compared with the creaking sound of old leather (Figure 5-23).

A distinctive feature of a pleural friction rub is that the sound audible during inspiration frequently recurs in reverse sequence during expiration. Forgacs refers to this as the "mirror image effect." Sometimes, the

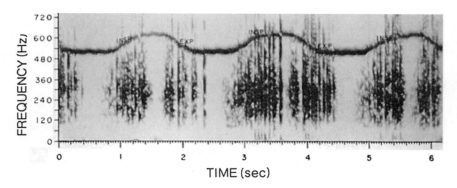

FIGURE 5-23. Pleural friction rub. Note the bursts of sound occurring in rapid succession. (From McKusick VA: *Cardiovascular sound in health and disease,* Baltimore, 1958, Williams & Wilkins.)

crackling sound made by a very high-pitched rub is indistinguishable from a crackle emanating from within the lung. In this case, differentiation is made on the basis of circumstantial evidence (Forgacs, 1978b); also, a rub is not affected by coughing.

Mediastinal Crunch (Hamman's Sign)

The mediastinal crunch is a coarse, crackling sound or vibration that is synchronous with systole and is frequently heard over the precordium in the presence of mediastinal emphysema. The air within the mediastinum producing the crunch may be present in trauma patients or patients who have undergone cardiopulmonary resuscitation. The distinctive crunching or popping sound is believed to result from air separating the visceral and parietal pericardium during contraction of the heart. Sometimes, the crunching also may be the result of left pneumothorax and gas in close contact with the heart or to elevation of the left hemidiaphragm caused by air in the fundus of the stomach.

According to Collins (1994), the rarity and dramatic nature of mediastinal crunch commonly result in an expensive evaluation and hospitalization. In fact, once recognized, a mediastinal crunch can be managed on an outpatient basis with serial chest radiographs to document resolution of the pneumomediastinum or pneumothorax.

Bronchial Leak Squeak

The bronchial leak squeak is a physical diagnostic sign in patients with bronchopleurocutaneous fistula. This sound is heard as a high-pitched squeak over the affected chest area during sustained Valsalva maneuver (expiration against a closed glottis), the pitch being higher in smaller fistulas than in larger fistulas. Decreases in intensity and increases in pitch occur in patients whose bronchial fistulas close slowly. When the leak squeak sign is absent in patients with spontaneous pneumothorax, one may assume that alveoli, rather than central airways, are leaking (Krumpe et al., 1981).

Inspiratory Squawk

A distinctive inspiratory musical sound, called a *squawk,* is found in some patients with diffuse pulmonary fibrosis (Earis et al., 1982). Allergic inflammation of the alveoli, also called *hypersensitivity pneumonitis,* appears to predispose to squawks.

Hypersensitivity pneumonitis results from the inhalation of organic antigens in susceptible individuals. The condition was initially described as "farmer's lung" and occurred after the inhalation of moldy hay contaminated by fungal organisms. Subsequently, many hobbies, occupations, and living conditions have been associated with this entity. Those affected include bird fanciers, detergent workers, mushroom pickers, cheese workers, and others. Maple bark, wood pulp, cork dust, coffee beans, redwood sawdust, and other substances have been demonstrated to cause the condition. Some substances may be contaminated by fungi, but often no fungus is involved.

Generally, the squawks of allergic alveolitis are of shorter duration, occur later in inspiration, and tend to be of higher pitch than those heard in pulmonary fibrosis of nonallergic origin. The squawk is almost invariably accompanied by inspiratory crackles. Like the crackles, the squawk seems to result from the opening of airways.

ABNORMALLY TRANSMITTED SOUNDS
Egophony

Egophony (Greek: *the voice of a goat*) refers to the nasal or bleating quality of speech transmitted through consolidated lung tissue (as, for example, in pneumonia) or occasionally over a pleural effusion, when the effusion causes collapse and atelectasis of underlying lung.

When voice sounds are transmitted to the chest wall through consolidated lung tissue, the normal sound filtering of the lung is diminished and, as a result, the higher frequencies are enhanced. Such a transmutation of the sound produces the phenomenon known as "E to A egophony" (McKusick, Jenkins, and Webb, 1955).

The raw material for speech, called the *voice source,* is the sound generated by the airstream chopped by the vocal cords. It is a complex tone comprising a fundamental frequency (determined by the vibratory frequency of the vocal cords) and a large number of higher-pitched harmonics, also called *overtones.*

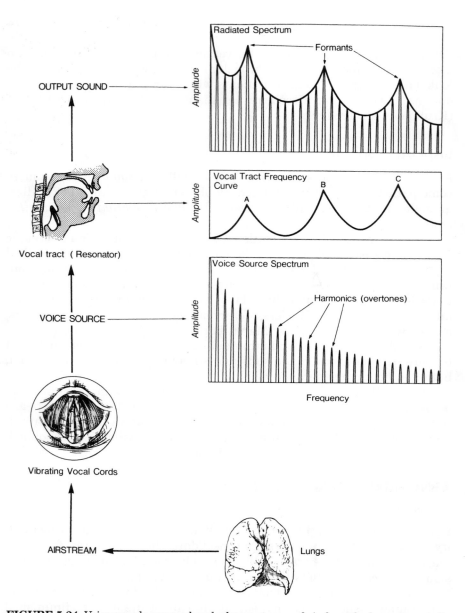

FIGURE 5-24. Voice sounds are produced when a stream of air from the lungs is periodically interrupted by the vibrating vocal cords. The resulting sound, the voice source, has a spectrum composed of a large number of harmonics, also called *overtones*. The vocal tract—the larynx, pharynx, nose, and mouth—is a resonator, that is, it has characteristic frequencies or formants (A, B, C) that it transmits best. As the voice source moves through the vocal tract, each harmonic is attenuated in proportion to its distance from the formant nearest it in frequency. The formant frequencies thus appear as peaks in the spectrum of sound radiated from the lips. The peaks establish particular vowel sounds. The higher peaks are not normally transmitted to the chest wall, thus rendering spoken words unintelligible through the stethoscope under ordinary conditions. However, the higher frequencies are transmitted through consolidated lung tissue in conditions such as pneumonia, rendering speech intelligible over the chest wall through a stethoscope. (Adapted from Sundberg J: *Sci Am* 236:82-91, 1977.)

The vocal tract—the larynx, pharynx, nose, and mouth—is a resonator; in other words, it has certain frequencies that it transmits best. The four or five most important of these frequencies are called *formants*. The closer a tone generated by the vocal cords is to the formant frequency, the louder it will be transmitted (Figure 5-24).

Figure 5-25 shows sound spectrograms of the letters *E* and *A* when spoken into a microphone. As can be seen, E lacks the higher frequencies or formants associated with A.

In Figure 5-26, the spectrogram on the left shows the normal letter *E* recorded through the chest wall. Notice the very prominent lowest formant at about 180 Hz. The spectrogram on the right shows the E to A

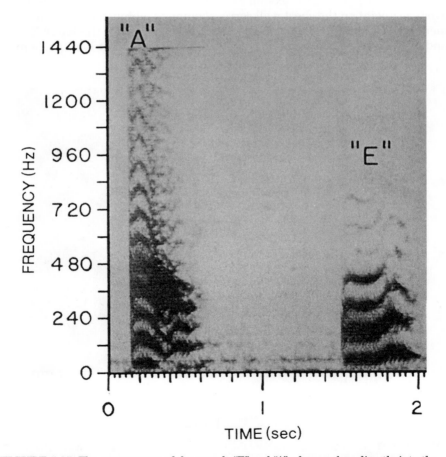

FIGURE 5-25. The spectrogram of the sounds "E" and "A" when spoken directly into the microphone. Note that "A" is composed of many more high-frequency components or formants than "E." (From McKusick VA, Jenkins JT, Webb GN: *Am Rev Tuberc* 72:12-34, 1955.)

change when heard through the consolidated lung of a patient with pneumonia. Notice that the upper frequencies have been enhanced, making the spoken E sound like A.

This phenomenon appears to have been discovered simultaneously in 1922, by Shibley in China (Shibley, 1922) and Froschels in Vienna (Froschels and Stockert, 1922). Shibley reported that five vowel sounds—A, E, I, O, U—all became "A" or "Ah," both over a localized area of fluid or consolidation and over a large goiter. He came upon the sign accidentally, while having his Chinese patients say "i, er, san" (one, two, three). The word for "one" was pronounced "E" in his province; thus the origin of the E to A sign. Froschels reported that one vowel sound might be changed into another with no particular predictability.

To elicit egophony, the examiner should place the bell of the stethoscope over each point on the chest wall corresponding to a bronchopulmonary segment (see Chapter 4). The patient should be asked to say the letter *E* over and over. If an "A"-like sound is perceived, then the patient has egophony.

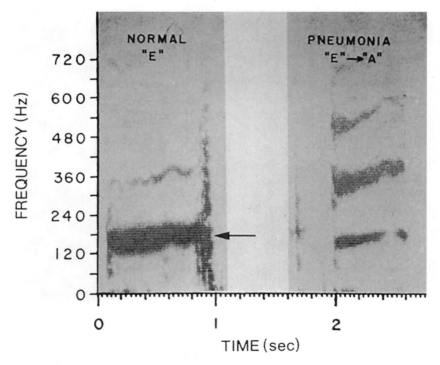

FIGURE 5-26. "E" to "A" egophony. Note the very prominent lowest formant of "E" *(arrow)* at about 180 Hz in the spectrogram on the left. The spectrogram on the right shows the "E" to "A" change when heard through the consolidated lung of a patient with pneumonia. Note that the higher frequencies have been enhanced, making the spoken "E" sound like "A." (From McKusick VA, Jenkins JT, Webb GN: *Am Rev Tuberc* 72:12-34, 1955.)

Whispered Pectoriloquy

During whispering, the vocal cords do not oscillate; voice sounds are generated by the turbulent flow of air through the trachea, glottis, and pharynx. This white noise is missing the prominent low-frequency oscillations (below 200 Hz) of normal voice sounds and is therefore much softer than normal speech.

Whispered sounds, which lack the low frequencies best transmitted by air-containing lung, are inaudible over the normal chest. However, through airless consolidated lung tissue, the high-pitched sounds (above 200 Hz) are transmitted, and the whispering becomes audible (Figure 5-27). This sign is called *whispered pectoriloquy.*

To elicit whispered pectoriloquy, the stethoscope should be placed over each bronchopulmonary segment. The patient should be asked to whisper "one, two, three." If the words are clearly audible over one segment, then the segment is designated as showing whispered pectoriloquy. The examiner should listen for whispered pectoriloquy with great care because, in general, it is more difficult to identify than other abnormal sounds, such as wheezing (Spitter, Cook, and Clarke, 1988).

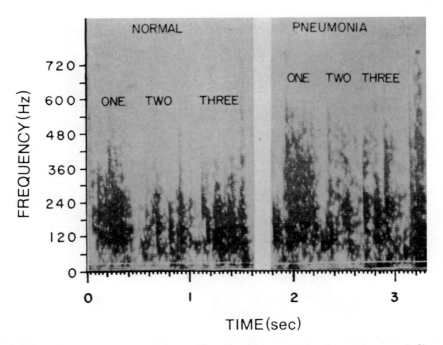

FIGURE 5-27. Whispered pectoriloquy. Note that in pneumonia, the spectrogram indicates that the higher frequencies in the words *one, two, three* have been transmitted, while in the normal subject they have not. The transmission of these higher frequencies makes the words intelligible through a stethoscope over the chest wall. (From McKusick VA, Jenkins JT, Webb GN: *Am Rev Tuberc* 72:12-34, 1955.)

Bronchophony and Bronchial Breathing

As the result of the selective transmission of sound through normal lung, the higher frequencies and most of the vowel formants are lost; speech heard through the stethoscope becomes a meaningless, low-pitched mumble. However, when lung between the stethoscope and the trachea is airless, the higher frequencies and vowel formants are transmitted. As a result speech becomes clear, a sign called *bronchophony*. Likewise, high-pitched breath sounds are transmitted through consolidated lung tissue to the chest wall in *bronchial breathing*.

Bronchophony and bronchial breathing are both signs of the unfiltered transmission of sounds through consolidated lung tissue; they are produced by the same mechanism as whispered pectoriloquy. For bronchial breathing to occur, consolidated lung tissue must extend at least 3 to 5 cm from the chest wall, except near the vertebral column, where it must be 1 to 2 cm from the surface (Martini and Muller, 1923; McKusick, Jenkins, and Webb, 1955).

To elicit bronchophony, the examiner should place the stethoscope over each bronchopulmonary segment. The patient should be asked to say

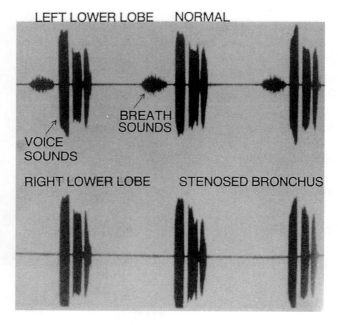

FIGURE 5-28. Simultaneous recordings of breath sounds and voice sounds at corresponding sites over the left lower lobe (normal bronchus) and right lower lobe (stenosed bronchus). Patient inspired deeply, spoke words "three, four, eight," and then exhaled. Three consecutive breaths are shown. Note that breath sounds are absent over the right lower lobe, which was stenosed. Note also that voice sounds were well transmitted on both sides. (From Jones FL: *Chest* 93:312-313, 1988.)

"ninety-nine." If these words are clearly audible and not a meaningless jumble, then bronchophony is said to be present.

Important note: All of the foregoing diagnostic signs—egophony, whispered pectoriloquy, bronchophony, and bronchial breathing—are the result of one thing: sound transmission through airless lung with resulting loss of normal filtering. They all have the same significance. Moreover, having the patient say "one, two, three" or "ninety-nine" is only a convention; in fact bronchophony and whispered pectoriloquy could be elicited just as well if the patient said almost anything.

Poor Breath Sounds with Good Voice Sounds

In patients with bronchial stenosis, the breath sounds over the involved lung are faint or absent, whereas the voice sounds are normal (Figure 5-28). This sign is applicable only to stenosis of the main, intermediate, or lobar bronchi (Jones, 1988).

Noisy Breathing at the Mouth

One of the most useful signs of chronic obstructive pulmonary disease is noisy breathing (Forgacs, 1978a). The breathing of most patients with chronic bronchitis or asthma is noisy, whereas the breath sounds of a healthy subject cannot be heard at a distance of a few centimeters from the mouth, unless he is panting, gasping, or sighing. The breathing of many patients with chronic obstructive pulmonary disease is accompanied by a noise that can be heard across the room. This noise is not to be confused with the adventitious sounds already discussed.

Forgacs has measured the noise during inspiration and confirmed the clinical observation that the loudness of the inspiratory breath sounds heard close to the patient's mouth reflects the severity of obstruction to the flow of air. The source of the noise appears to be turbulence in the gas flowing through the airways.

RELATIONSHIP OF BREATH SOUND INTENSITY TO VENTILATORY FUNCTION

Since the nineteenth century, medical writings have referred to a reduction in the loudness of breath sounds over the chest as evidence for the presence of emphysema. This observation has been tested on a quantitative basis by Pardee and associates (1976) and Bohadana and colleagues (1978). Diminished breath sounds correlated quite well with diminished percentage of predicted forced expiratory volume in one second (FEV_1) and with other measurements of obstruction and vital capacity. In other words, patients with emphysema and very faint breath sounds will probably have very poor pulmonary function. Indeed, patients with severe emphysema often have practically no detectable lung sounds at all.

A useful, quantitative way to test for the loudness of breath sounds is by obtaining a breath sound score. To obtain this score, auscultation is performed at the following six locations: bilaterally over the upper anterior portion of the chest, in the midaxillae, and at the posterior bases. Breath sound intensity is estimated in inspiration during a response to the request that the subject take a deep breath with his mouth open. The loudness of the sounds is scaled in five stages: 0—silent, 1—barely audible, 2—faint but definitely heard breath sounds, 3—expected for normal, and 4—louder than usual normal. The numeric grades for the six areas sampled are added to give a total breath sound score. The score can then be compared with the following table to obtain a crude approximation of FEV_1/FVC (see Chapter 1 for the significance of this measurement):

Total Breath Sound Score	FEV₁/FVC (%)
10	27
12	38
14	49
16	60
18	71
20	82

Example: A 55-year-old white man, a heavy smoker, was examined. The examiner obtained the following scores:

Location	Breath Sound Score
Right upper anterior chest	3
Left upper anterior chest	2
Right midaxilla	2
Left midaxilla	3
Right posterior base	3
Left posterior base	1
Total breath sound score	14

From the table, the patient has an FEV_1/FVC of 49%.

SLEEP APNEA SYNDROME

During sleep persons with sleep apnea periodically stop breathing. Many normal people stop breathing 10 times a night or less for a period of less than 20 seconds. However a person with sleep apnea may stop breathing once or twice every minute; this adds up to almost 1000 apneas over 8 hours, each of which may last from 10 to more than 60 seconds.

Patients with sleep apnea complain most commonly of excessive daytime sleepiness, but they also may note insomnia. A spouse or bedmate will complain of their loud, excessive snoring. Sleep apnea may be classified as two types, obstructive and nonobstructive.

Obstructive sleep apnea is the result of a periodic obstruction within the upper airway, usually in an obese male with a thick neck. The definitive treatment for this condition is a tracheostomy, which creates a bypass below the upper airway obstruction. For obstructive sleep apneas that are not severe enough to warrant a tracheostomy, one experimental form of treatment is the placement of a mask that fits over the face and is worn at night to provide a positive pressure on the airway and thus keep it open.

Nonobstructive sleep apnea results from an abnormality of the respiratory center in the pons, a section of the brain near the medulla. The abnormality may be the result of vascular disease, meningitis, encephalitis, or tumor or may be of unknown cause. Breathing is normal, without apnea, in the patient who is awake, because the inadequacy of the respiratory center is compensated for by other impulses moving through the cortical tracts of the brain. However, during sleep, when cortical impulses cease, the respiratory center is insufficient to maintain regular respiration. Tracheostomy is of no value in nonobstructive sleep apnea.

To differentiate obstructive from nonobstructive sleep apnea, airflow at the nose and mouth and respiratory effort are assessed. Respiratory effort is gauged with a chest strain gauge, intercostal electromyogram, intraesophageal balloon, and other devices. Airflow is sometimes estimated by recording tracheal breath sounds. If respiratory effort is normal while no airflow is detected, then the apnea is of obstructive origin. If there is no airflow and no muscular activity, then the apnea is nonobstructive (Cummiskey et al., 1982; Kupfer and Reynolds, 1983).

A diagrammatic summary of common adventitious breath sounds is presented in Figure 5-29.

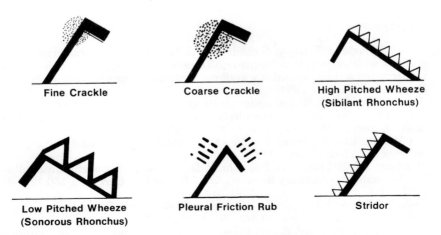

Fine Crackle   Coarse Crackle   High Pitched Wheeze (Sibilant Rhonchus)

Low Pitched Wheeze (Sonorous Rhonchus)   Pleural Friction Rub   Stridor

FIGURE 5-29. Diagrammatic summary of common adventitious breath sounds.

Chapter Review and Critical Thinking Questions

1. *What is a crackle? What is the cause of crackling?*

2. *Name and describe the types of disease associated with (a) early inspiratory crackles and (b) late inspiratory crackles.*

3. *What is a wheeze? What is the correct mechanism of wheezing?*

4. *What is the difference between a monophonic wheeze and a polyphonic wheeze?*

5. *What is stridor? Name and describe the conditions commonly associated with stridor, both in children and in adults.*

6. *What pathologic condition is associated with a mediastinal crunch?*

7. *What is the pathologic significance of an inspiratory "squawk"?*

8. *What is heard in a patient with egophony? What pathologic conditions are associated with egophony? Describe the sound transmutation that produces egophony.*

9. *Describe whispered pectoriloquy. With what pathologic conditions is it associated?*

10. *Describe bronchophony and bronchial breathing. With what pathologic conditions are they associated?*

11. *What effect does emphysema have on the amplitude of breath sounds heard over the chest?*

12. *What is the significance of crackles heard over the chest after a myocardial infarction, while the patient is still in the coronary care unit?*

BIBLIOGRAPHY

al Jarad N, Davies SW, Logan-Sinclair R et al: Lung crackle characteristics in patients with asbestosis, asbestos-related pleural disease, and left ventricular failure using a time-expanded waveform analysis—a comparative study, *Respir Med* 88:37-46, 1994.

al Jarad N, Strickland B, Bothamley G: Diagnosis of asbestosis by a time expanded waveform analysis, auscultation and high resolution computed tomography: a comparative study, *Thorax* 48:347-353, 1993.

Beers MH, Berkow R, editors: *The Merck manual of diagnosis and therapy,* Rahway, NJ, 1999, Merck.

Bettencourt PE, Del Bono EA, Spiegelman D: Clinical utility of chest auscultation in common pulmonary diseases, *Am J Respir Crit Care Med* 150:1291-1297, 1994.

Bohadana AB, Peslin R, Uffholtz H: Breath sounds in the clinical assessment of airflow obstruction, *Thorax* 33:345-351, 1978.

Christopher KL, Wood RP, Eckert RC et al: Vocal cord dysfunction presenting as asthma, *N Engl J Med* 308:1566-1570, 1983.

Collins RK: Hamman's crunch: an adventitious sound, *J Fam Pract* 38:284-286, 1994.

Cugell DW: Sounds of the lungs, *Chest* 73:311-312, 1978.

Cummiskey J, Williams TC, Krumpe PE et al: The detection and quantification of sleep apnea by tracheal sound recordings, *Am Rev Respir Dis* 126:221-224, 1982.

Deguchi F, Hirakawa S, Gotoh K: Prognostic significance of posturally induced crackles. Long-term follow-up of patients after recovery from acute myocardial infarction, *Chest* 103:1457-1462, 1993.

Earis JE, Marsh K, Pearson MG et al: The inspiratory "squawk" in extrinsic allergic alveolitis and other pulmonary fibroses, *Thorax* 37:923-926, 1982.

Epler GR, Carrington CB, Gaensler EA: Crackles (rales) in the interstitial pulmonary diseases, *Chest* 73:333-339, 1978.

Forgacs P: The functional basis of pulmonary sounds, *Chest* 73:399-405, 1978a.

Forgacs P: *Lung sounds,* London, 1978b, Baillière Tindall.

Froschels E, Stockert FG: Über ein neues Symptom bei Lungen und Pleurakrankheiten, *Wien Klin Wochenschr* 35:500, 1922.

Hudson LD, Conn RD, Matsubara RS et al: Rales: diagnostic uselessness of qualitative adjectives, *Am Rev Respir Dis* 113:187, 1976.

Jones AY, Jones RD, Kwong K: The effect on sound generation of varying both gas flow rate and the viscosity of sputum-like gel in a simple tubular model, *Lung* 178:31-40, 2000.

Jones FL: Poor breath sounds with good voice sounds: a sign of bronchial stenosis, *Chest* 93:312-313, 1988.

Kraman SS: The forced expiratory wheeze: its site of origin and possible association with lung compliance, *Respiration* 44:189-196, 1983.

Kraman SS: Lung sounds for the clinician, *Arch Intern Med* 146:1411-1412, 1986.

Krumpe P, Finley T, Wong L et al: The bronchial leak squeak: a new sign for the physical diagnosis of bronchopleurocutaneous fistula, *Chest* 79:336-339, 1981.

Kupfer DJ, Reynolds CF: Sleep disorders, *Hosp Pract* 18:101-124, 1983.

Ludman H: Hoarseness and stridor, *BMJ* 282:715-717, 1981.

Martini P, Müller H: Studien über das Bronchialatmen, *Dtsch Arch Klin Med* 143:159-173, 1923.

McKusick VA, Jenkins JT, Webb GN: The acoustic basis of the chest examination: studies by means of sound spectrography, *Am Rev Tuberc* 72:12-34, 1955.

Mikami R, Murao M, Cugell D et al: International symposium on lung sounds: synopsis of proceedings, *Chest* 92:342-345, 1987.

Mori M, Kinoshita K, Morinari H et al: Waveform and spectral analysis of crackles, *Thorax* 35:843-850, 1980.

Multicenter Postinfarction Research Group: Risk stratification and survival after myocardial infarction, *N Engl J Med* 309:331-336, 1983.

Munakata M, Ukita H, Doi I et al: Spectral and waveform characteristics of fine and coarse crackles, *Thorax* 46:651-657, 1991.

Murphy RL: Auscultation of the lung: past lessons, future possibilities, *Thorax* 36:99-107, 1981.

Nath AR, Capel LH: Inspiratory crackles—early and late, *Thorax* 29:223-227, 1974a.

Nath AR, Capel LH: Inspiratory crackles and mechanical events of breathing, *Thorax* 29:695-698, 1974b.

Nath AR, Capel LH: Lung crackles in bronchiectasis, *Thorax* 35:694-699, 1980.

Pardee NE, Martin CJ, Morgan EH: A test of the practical value of estimating breath sound intensity: breath sounds related to measured ventilatory function, *Chest* 70:341-344, 1976.

Pasterkamp H, Montgomery M, Wiebicke W: Nomenclature used by health care professionals to describe breath sounds in asthma, *Chest* 92:346-352, 1987.

Pasterkamp H, Wiebicke W, Fenton R: Subjective assessment vs. computer analysis of wheezing in asthma, *Chest* 91:376-381, 1987.

Roberts KB, editor: *Manual of clinical problems in pediatrics,* Boston, 1979, Little, Brown.

Robertson JA, Cope R: Rales, rhonchi, and Laennec, *Lancet* 2:417, 1957.

Sapira JD: About egophony, *Chest* 108:865-867, 1995.

Say ninety-nine, *Lancet* 2:1258-1259, 1986 (editorial).

Shibley GS: New auscultatory sign found in consolidation, or collection of fluid in pulmonary disease, *Chin Med J* 36:1, 1922.

Shirai F, Kudoh S, Shibuya A et al: Crackles in asbestos workers: auscultation and lung sound analysis, *Br J Dis Chest* 75:386-396, 1981.

Spitter MA, Cook DG, Clarke SW: Reliability of eliciting physical signs in examination of the chest, *Lancet* 1:873-875, 1988.

Thacker R, Kraman SS: The incidence of auscultatory crackles in subjects without lung disease, *Chest* 81:672-674, 1982.

Workum P, Holford S, del Bono E et al: The prevalence of crackles in young adult females, *Am Rev Respir Dis* 126:921, 1982.

Answer Guidelines for Chapter Review and Critical Thinking Questions

Chapter 1. Anatomy, Physiology, and Pathophysiology Review

1. The trachea divides into the right and left main bronchi at the carina. The right bronchus leaves the bifurcation at less of an angle than does the left bronchus; for this reason, aspirated fluids are more prone to enter the right lung.

2. Gas in the alveoli does not contact the alveolar epithelium directly; instead, the surface is covered by a layer of fluid containing a substance called **surfactant,** which imparts the lowest surface tension of any biologic material ever tested. Low surface tension at this location is important; it keeps alveoli from collapsing. When surfactant is deficient, as in the neonatal respiratory distress syndrome, atelectasis and severe mechanical disturbances occur. Surfactant is a phospholipid that is secreted by special cells of the alveolar epithelium.

3. Normal inspiratory breathing at rest is performed by contraction of the muscles of inspiration—the diaphragm and external intercostals. Normal expiration is passive and requires no muscular effort because it results from elastic recoil of the lung and thorax.

4. A typical **spirometer** consists of a drum inverted over a chamber of water, with the drum counterbalanced by a weight (Figure 1-5). The drum contains a breathing mixture of gases, usually air or oxygen; the mouth is connected to the gas chamber by a tube. When the subject breathes in and out of the chamber, the drum rises and falls, and a recording is made on a moving sheet of paper.

5. Among the **restrictive** lung diseases are advanced tuberculosis and silicosis; diffuse interstitial pulmonary fibrosis of unknown etiology; kyphosis and scoliosis, which constrict the chest cage; drug-induced fibrotic reactions; and fibrosis secondary to chemical or physical injury.

6. A simple, useful test of airway obstruction is the *forced expiratory vital capacity* (FVC). Recordings of FVC are made on a spirometer. To obtain the recording, the examiner asks the subject to inspire maximally to total lung capacity, then to exhale into the spirometer with maximum expiratory effort as rapidly and completely as possible. The total excursion of the record represents the FVC.

7. Any of the following abnormalities tend to diminish the **vital capacity:**
   A. *Paralysis of the respiratory muscles.* This often occurs after spinal cord injuries or poliomyelitis and can decrease vital capacity 1000 to 500 ml.
   B. *Diminished pulmonary compliance ("stiff lungs").* Tuberculosis, lung cancer, and pulmonary fibrosis can all reduce pulmonary compliance and thereby decrease vital capacity.

C. Pulmonary vascular congestion. In left-sided heart failure or any other condition causing pulmonary vascular congestion and edema, vital capacity is reduced because excess fluid in the lungs decreases compliance.

Chapter 2. Sound, Hearing, and the Stethoscope

1. Sound has three principal characteristics: frequency, intensity, and duration.

A. Frequency is a measure of the number of vibrations per unit time, in cycles per second or hertz (Hz). A large number of vibrations, as in a high-frequency wheeze, yields a sound that is subjectively interpreted by the examiner as being high-pitched. A low-frequency wheeze, on the other hand, gives a sound that is heard as low-pitched.

B. Intensity is governed by four factors: (1) the amplitude of the vibrations, (2) the source producing the energy, (3) the distance the vibrations must travel, and (4) the medium through which they travel. These factors determine whether a sound is perceived as loud or faint. For example, breath sounds are much fainter than normal over an emphysematous lung because the damaged, hyperaerated tissue conducts sound poorly.

C. Duration of the vibrations determines whether the ear interprets them as short or long, for example, a short wheeze or a long wheeze.

2. *Sound quality,* also known as *timbre,* is determined by the component frequencies that make up any particular sound.

3. A wheeze is analogous to a musical note.

4. Most breath sounds are more difficult to perceive than other types of sound because they fall into a frequency range to which the ear is relatively insensitive.

5. The open bell, or Ford chest piece, is similar to the old-fashioned trumpet-type hearing aid. It conducts sounds with practically no distortion. The bell is well suited for listening to low-pitched sounds. The closed diaphragm, or Bowles chest piece, has a larger diameter than the bell. The diaphragm is best suited for hearing high-pitched sounds because it acts to attenuate low-frequency sounds and pass high-frequency sounds.

Chapter 3. History and Physical Examination

1. The **chief complaint** is the problem and the duration of the problem, that causes the patient to seek medical attention, such as cough, shortness of breath, abnormal chest radiograph on routine physical examination.

2. **Occupational history** is important because both acute and chronic respiratory disease may result from certain types of dust inhaled at work.

3. The caregiver should specifically inquire about past history of tuberculosis, pneumonia, and chest injuries.

4. The two types of cough are productive (i.e., of sputum) and nonproductive (i.e., dry cough).

5. Bronchiectasis and active pulmonary tuberculosis are frequently associated with massive hemoptysis.

Chapter 4. Normal Breath Sounds

1. The four types of breath sounds audible over the normal chest are the following:

A. Normal vesicular. This is a relatively soft, low-pitched sound, sometimes described as a sighing or gentle rustling; it is heard over most of the peripheral parts of the lung. The inspiratory phase is markedly longer than the expiratory phase, with the I:E ratio being about 3:1. Expiration is much quieter than inspiration, usually being almost inaudible. There is no pause between inspiration and expiration.

B. Bronchial. These characteristically loud, high-pitched sounds resemble the sound of air blowing through a hollow pipe. Their expiratory phase is louder and longer than their inspiratory phase. They are normally present only over the manubrium, and a distinct pause can be heard between the inspiratory and expiratory phases.

C. Bronchovesicular. These sounds are a mixture of bronchial and vesicular sounds. Their inspiratory and expiratory phases are about equal in length (I:E ratio = 1:1). They are normally audible in two places: (1) anteriorly, near the mainstem bronchi in the first and second intercostal spaces; and (2) posteriorly, between the scapulae. To hear them elsewhere may mean lung consolidation or another abnormality.

D. Tracheal. These sounds, not usually auscultated, are present over the extrathoracic portion of the trachea. They are very loud, very high-pitched, and have a hollow or harsh quality. The expiratory phase is slightly longer than the inspiratory phase.

2. Normal vesicular breath sounds are produced by turbulent air flow in the larger airways.

3. In a normal individual in the upright position, breath sounds at the lung apex become progressively fainter during inspiration from residual volume. In contrast, at the lung base, the breath sounds are relatively faint at the beginning of inspiration; their intensity increases to a maximum at 50% of the vital capacity.

4. In some healthy individuals, breath sounds over the left lower lobe rise and fall in synchrony with the heartbeat. Usually, they are loud-

est during systole, when contraction of the ventricles allows the adjacent lung tissue to expand, lowering alveolar pressure and facilitating gas flow into the left lower lobe.

5. Sounds at the mouth are different from sounds heard through the chest wall because of the different paths of transmission. Breath sounds at the mouth consist of a broad range of evenly distributed frequencies between 200 and 2000 cycles. In contrast, the chest wall and lung act as so-called low pass filters and allow only the low frequencies to pass through.

6. Breath sounds transmitted through the chest fade out during expiration, whereas those over the trachea can be heard throughout the respiratory cycle. The following two reasons account for this discrepancy:

A. Although rate of air flow falls continuously during expiration, the breath sounds over the trachea are so loud that they remain above the threshold of hearing throughout the respiratory cycle. The sounds transmitted through the chest wall are much fainter, and they contain mostly low frequencies, to which the ear is less sensitive. Thus the breath sounds become too soft to hear early in expiration.

B. During inspiration, turbulence is most likely generated and carried farther toward the periphery of the lung than during expiration. Because the turbulence moves away from the chest wall during expiration, the resulting faint breath sounds are absorbed by the lung before they reach the stethoscope.

7. Laryngeal sounds do not contribute to the normal vesicular breath sounds. The amplitude of the simultaneously recorded vesicular sounds correlates only with flow rates and is completely unaffected by changes in laryngeal sound amplitude.

Chapter 5. Abnormal Breath Sounds

1. *Crackles* are short, explosive, nonmusical sounds. The most widely accepted cause of crackling is the explosive equalization of gas pressure between two compartments of the lung, when a closed section of the airways separating them suddenly opens.

2. *Early inspiratory crackles* are characteristic of patients with severe airway obstruction and the following conditions: chronic bronchitis, asthma, and emphysema. *Late inspiratory crackles* are characteristic of patients with restrictive pulmonary disease and the following conditions: interstitial fibrosis, asbestosis, pneumonia, pulmonary congestion of heart failure, pulmonary sarcoidosis, scleroderma, and rheumatoid lung.

3. A *wheeze* (rhonchus) is a musical pulmonary sound. The most widely accepted mechanism of wheezing is analogous to a vibrating reed.

4. A monophonic wheeze is a single musical tone. A polyphonic wheeze is confined largely to expiration and is composed of several dissonant notes starting and ending at the same time.

5. *Stridor* is a particularly loud musical sound of constant pitch, most prominent during inspiration, and heard very well at a distance from the patient. In children, stridor is often the result of laryngomalacia, viral croup, acute epiglottitis, diphtheria, laryngeal paralysis, congenital narrowing of the larynx or trachea, or inhalation of a foreign body. In adults, stridor may result from chronic laryngitis, vocal cord paralysis, or tumors of the larynx.

6. *Mediastinal crunch* may be present in trauma patients or patients who have undergone cardiopulmonary resuscitation. Sometimes, the crunching may also be the result of left-sided pneumothorax and gas in close contact with the heart, or to elevation of the left hemidiaphragm caused by air in the fundus of the stomach.

7. *Inspiratory squawk* is found in some patients with diffuse pulmonary fibrosis. Allergic inflammation of the alveoli, also called *hypersensitivity pneumonitis,* also predisposes to squawks.

8. *Egophony* is the nasal or bleating quality of speech transmitted through consolidated lung tissue (as, for example, in pneumonia) or occasionally over a pleural effusion, when the effusion causes collapse and atelectasis of underlying lung. When voice sounds are transmitted to the chest wall through consolidated lung tissue, the normal sound filtering of the lung is diminished and, as a result, the higher frequencies are enhanced. Such a transmutation of the sound produces the phenomenon known as *E to A egophony.*

9. Whispered sounds, which lack the low frequencies best transmitted by air-containing lung, are inaudible over the normal chest. However, through airless consolidated lung tissue, the high-pitched whispered sounds (above 200 Hz) are transmitted, and the whispering becomes audible. This sign is called *whispered pectoriloquy.*

10. As the result of the selective transmission of sound through normal lung, the higher frequencies and most of the vowel formants are lost. Speech heard through the stethoscope becomes a meaningless, low pitched mumble. However, when lung between the stethoscope and the trachea is airless, the higher frequencies and vowel formants are transmitted. As a result speech becomes clear, a sign called *bronchophony.* Likewise, high-pitched breath sounds are transmitted through consolidated lung tissue to the chest wall in *bronchial breathing.* Bronchophony and bronchial breathing are both signs of the unfiltered transmission of sounds through consolidated lung tissue; they are produced by the same mechanism as whispered pectoriloquy.

11. Emphysema reduces the amplitude of breath sounds heard over the chest.

12. *Crackles after a myocardial infarct* that appear over the upper two thirds of the posterior lung fields, while the patient is still in the coronary care unit, are an extremely bad sign. A patient with such crackles is 3.3 times more likely to die in the 2-year period following the infarct than is the same patient without these crackles. Crackles heard only at the lung bases—that is, the lower third of the posterior lung fields—do not have the same dire significance.

GLOSSARY

Achalasia: Failure of the smooth muscle fibers of the gastrointestinal tract to relax at any point of junction of one part with another. An example is the failure of the smooth muscle fibers of the lower esophagus to relax, called *achalasia of the esophagus,* which is characterized by dilation and hypertrophy of the esophagus above an atrophic lower segment (megaesophagus).

Adduction: A drawing together.

Aneurysm: A sac formed by the dilation of the walls of an artery or of a vein filled with blood. A dissecting aneurysm is one in which the blood is forced between the coats of an artery.

Angina pectoris: A paroxysmal thoracic pain, with a feeling of suffocation and impending death. This is usually the result of insufficient oxygen reaching the heart muscle and is precipitated by effort or excitement.

Antigen: A high molecular weight substance or complex, usually protein or protein polysaccharide in nature. When it is foreign to the blood stream of an animal, on gaining access to the tissues of such an animal it stimulates the formation of a specific antibody and reacts specifically in vivo or in vitro with its homologous antibody.

Aorta: The main trunk from which the systemic arterial system proceeds. It arises from the left ventricle of the heart, passes upward, bends over, and passes down through the thorax and abdomen to the fourth lumbar vertebra, where it divides into the two common iliac arteries.

Apex (pulmonary): The rounded upper extremity of either lung, extending upward as high as the first thoracic vertebra; also called *lung apex.*

Apnea: The transient cessation of breathing.

Arytenoids: A pair of ladle-shaped cartilages that form part of the larynx.

Asbestos: A fibrous magnesium and calcium silicate often used for thermal insulation.

Ascites: Effusion of serous fluid into the abdominal cavity.

Atelectasis: Incomplete expansion or collapse of the lung.

Atrophy: A defect or failure of nutrition manifested as a wasting away or diminution in the size of a cell, tissue, organ, or part.

Axilla: The small hollow beneath the arm, where it joins the body at the shoulder; also called *armpit.*

Binaural: Pertaining to both ears.

Biopsy: The removal and examination, usually microscopic, of tissue or other material from the living body for purposes of diagnosis.

Bronchiectasis: A chronic dilation of the bronchi or bronchioles.

Bronchiole: One of the finer subdivisions of the branched bronchial tree.

Bronchitis: An inflammation of the bronchial tubes.

Bronchophony: The sound of the voice as heard through the stethoscope applied over a healthy bronchus. When heard elsewhere, it indicates solidification of the lung tissue.

Bronchopleural: Pertaining to a bronchus and the pleura, or communicating with a bronchus and the pleural cavity, as a bronchopleural fistula.

Bronchus: One of the larger air passages within the lungs.

Bulla: In the lung, a bubble-shaped abnormality often associated with emphysema.

Carina: A keel-shaped structure, a projection of the lowest tracheal cartilage, which forms a prominent semilunar ridge running anteroposteriorly between the orifices of the two bronchi.

Cochlea: The essential organ of hearing, a spiral-wound tube that resembles a snail shell and forms part of the inner ear.

Consolidation: Solidification, as of a lung in pneumonia.

Costochondral: Pertaining to a rib and its cartilage.

Crackle: A short, explosive, nonmusical sound heard over the chest, and sometimes at the mouth.

Crepitation: A crackling noise, as would be made when there is air in subcutaneous tissue or when the ends of fractured bones rub together.

Cyanosis: A bluish discoloration of skin and mucous membranes resulting from excessive concentration of reduced hemoglobin in the blood.

Diaphragm: The musculomembranous partition separating the abdominal and thoracic cavities.

Diastole: The dilation, or period of dilation, of the heart, especially that of the ventricles. It coincides with the interval between the second and first heart sounds.

Dyspnea: Difficult or labored breathing.

Edema: Swelling.

Effusion: The escape of fluid into a part or tissue.

Egophony: A bleating quality of voice observed in auscultation in certain cases of lung consolidation.

Embolus: A clot or other plug carried by the blood from another vessel and forced into a smaller one so as to obstruct the circulation.

Emphysema: A swelling or inflation as a result of the presence of air. This applies especially to a pathologic condition of the lungs, pulmonary emphysema, in which there is an increase beyond normal in the size of air spaces distal to the terminal bronchioles, either from dilation of the alveoli or from destruction of their walls.

Empyema: Accumulation of pus in a cavity of the body, especially in the chest (pyothorax).

Encephalitis: Inflammation of the brain.

Epiglottis: An elastic cartilage, covered by mucous membrane, that forms the upper part of the larynx and guards the glottis during swallowing.

Esophagus: The musculomembranous passage extending from the pharynx to the stomach.

Etiology: Cause.

Fibrosis: The formation of fibrous tissue.

Fistula: An abnormal passage or communication, usually between two internal organs, or leading from an internal organ to the surface of the body. It is frequently designated according to the organs or parts with which it communicates, for example, bronchocutaneous.

Fremitus: A thrill or vibration, especially one that is perceptible on palpation.

Glottis: The vocal apparatus of the larynx, consisting of the true vocal cords (vocal folds) and the opening between them (*rima glottidis*).

Goiter: An enlargement of the thyroid gland, causing a swelling in the front part of the neck.

Granuloma: A localized nodule of inflammatory tissue showing the process of granulation. A caseating granuloma is associated with tuberculosis; a noncaseating granuloma is seen in sarcoidosis.

Hematemesis: The vomiting of blood.
Hemoptysis: The coughing up of blood or blood-stained sputum.
Hemothorax: Blood in the pleural space.
Hiatus hernia: Protrusion of any structure through the esophageal hiatus of the diaphragm.
Hilum: The recess in the lung just above the cardiac impression.
Hypertrophy: The morbid enlargement or overgrowth of an organ or part because of an increase in size of its constituent cells.

Idiopathic: Of unknown cause.
Intensity: An objective assessment of sound, determined by the amplitude of the vibrations, their generating source, the distance traveled, and the medium through which they travel.
Intercostal: Situated between the ribs.
Intubation: The insertion of a tube into the airway to facilitate breathing.

Kyphosis: A condition characterized by an abnormally increased convexity in the curvature of the thoracic spine as viewed from the side; also called a *humpback.*

Larynx: The musculocartilaginous structure, lined with mucous membrane, situated at the top of the trachea and below the root of the tongue and the hyoid bone. It is the essential sphincter guarding the entrance into the trachea and functions secondarily as the organ of the voice.

Mediastinum: The mass of tissues and organs separating the two lungs between the sternum in front and the vertebral column behind and from the thoracic inlet above to the diaphragm below. It contains the heart and its large vessels, as well as the trachea, esophagus, thymus, lymph nodes, and other structures and tissues. It is divided into anterior, middle, posterior, and superior regions.

Meningitis: An inflammation of the meninges, the three membranes (dura mater, pia mater, and arachnoid) that envelop the brain and the spinal cord.
Mesothelioma: A primary tumor of the cells forming the lining of the peritoneum, pericardium, or pleura.
Mitral stenosis: Narrowing of the left atrioventricular orifice.
Mycoplasma: A taxonomic name given a genus including the pleuropneumonia-like organisms (PPLO), and separated into 15 species on the basis of source, glucose fermentation, and growth on agar media.
Myocardial infarction: An area of coagulation necrosis in the heart muscle as a result of an interruption of the blood supply to that area.

Nasopharynx: That part of the pharynx above the level of the soft palate, communicating with the posterior nares and the auditory tube.
Neoplastic: Pertaining to a new and abnormal growth, such as a tumor.
Neuritis: Inflammation of a nerve.
Noncaseating: A degenerative change not having the consistency of cheese.

Oncotic: Pertaining to, caused by, or marked by swelling.
Orthopnea: The need to sit up in order to avoid breathing difficulty; associated with heart disease.

Paroxysm: A sudden recurrence or intensification of symptoms.
Pectoriloquy: Transmission of the sound of spoken words through the chest wall. Whispered pectoriloquy is the transmission of the sound of whispered words through the chest wall and indicates lung consolidation.

Pericardium: The fibroserous sac that surrounds the heart, comprising an external layer of dense fibrous tissue (fibrous pericardium) and an inner serous layer (serous pericardium). The visceral pericardium is the inner layer of the serous pericardium in contact with the heart. The parietal pericardium is that layer in contact with the fibrous pericardium.

Peritoneum: The serous membrane lining the abdominopelvic walls and investing the viscera.

pH: The symbol commonly used in expressing hydrogen ion concentration, the measure of alkalinity and acidity. It signifies the logarithm of the reciprocal of the hydrogen ion concentration in gram molecules per liter of solution. A pH of 7 is the neutral point; greater than 7, alkalinity increases; less than 7, acidity increases.

Pharynx: The musculomembranous sac between the mouth and nares and the esophagus. It is continuous below with the esophagus, and above it communicates with the larynx, mouth, nasal passages, and auditory tubes.

Pleura: The serous membrane investing the lungs and lining the thoracic cavity, completely enclosing a potential space known as the pleural cavity. The parietal pleura is that portion lining the walls of the thoracic cavity. The visceral pleura is that portion investing the lungs and lining their fissures, completely separating the different lobes.

Pneumothorax: An accumulation of air in the pleural cavity, which may occur spontaneously or as a result of trauma, a pathologic process, or deliberate induction.

Precordium: The region over the heart or stomach; the epigastrium and lower part of the thorax.

Prodrome: A premonitory symptom or precursor; a symptom indicating the onset of a disease.

Psittacosis: A microbial disease first observed in parrots and known to be communicated by them to man and later discovered to exist in other birds and domestic fowl.

Purulent: Consisting of or containing pus.

Resonance: The prolongation and intensification of sound produced by the transmission of its vibrations to a cavity.

Rhonchus: A musical pulmonary sound (also called a *wheeze*).

Scoliosis: An appreciable lateral deviation in the normally straight vertical line of the spine.

Sibilant: High-pitched.

Sonorous: Low-pitched.

Sphincter: A ring-like band of muscle fibers that constricts a passage or closes a natural orifice.

Sputum: Matter ejected from the lungs, bronchi, and trachea through the mouth.

Stenosis: A narrowing.

Sternum: A longitudinal unpaired plate of bone forming the middle of the anterior wall of the thorax. It articulates above with the clavicles and along the sides with the cartilages of the first seven ribs and consists of three portions: the manubrium, the body, and the xiphoid process.

Syncope: A sudden loss of strength; a temporary suspension of consciousness resulting from cerebral anemia; a faint.

Systole: The contraction, or period of contraction, of the heart, especially the ventricles. It corresponds with the interval between the first and second heart sounds, during which the blood is forced into the aorta and pulmonary trunk.

Thorax: The part of the body between the neck and the respiratory diaphragm, encased by the ribs; the chest.

Thyroidectomy: Removal of part or all of the thyroid gland.

Tomography: A special x-ray technique to show detail in images of structures lying in a predetermined plane of tissue, while blurring or eliminating detail in images of structures in other planes. It is also called *body section roentgenography.*

Trachea: The cartilaginous and membranous tube descending from the larynx to the bronchi.

Tracheostomy: Surgical creation of an opening into the trachea through the neck for insertion of a tube to facilitate the passage of air into the lungs or for the evacuation of secretions.

Unilateral: One-sided.

Valsalva maneuver: Expiratory effort against a closed glottis.

Varices (plural of varix): Enlarged and tortuous vessels. Esophageal varices are enlarged and tortuous veins.

Viscosity: A physical property of a substance that is dependent on the friction of its component molecules as they slide by one another. For example, cold maple syrup is more viscous than water.

Wheeze: A musical pulmonary sound (also called a *rhonchus*).

INDEX

An "f" following a page number indicates a figure; a "t" indicates a table.

Abdominal muscles, 5
Abnormal breath sounds, 87-124. *See also* Normal breath sounds.
   abnormally transmitted sounds, 113-119
   adventitious sounds, 88-113
   airway obstruction, 111
   bronchial breathing, 118
   bronchial leak squeak, 112-113
   bronchial stenosis, 119
   bronchophony, 118-119
   crackles, 88-100. *See also* Crackles.
   croup, 106
   diphtheria, 106-107
   egophony, 113-116
   epiglottitis, 106
   hoarseness, 108-110
   inspiratory squawk, 113
   laryngitis, 108
   laryngomalcia, 105-106
   loudness of breath sounds, 119-120
   mediastinal crunch, 112
   neoplasms of larynx, 109-110
   noisy breathing, 119
   pleural friction rub, 111-112
   poor breath sounds/good voice sounds, 119
   sleep apnea, 120-121
   stridor, 105-108
   terminology, 87-88
   vocal cord paralysis, 108-109
   wheezes, 100-105. *See also* Wheezes.
   whispered pectoriloquy, 117
Abnormally transmitted sounds
   bronchial breathing, 118
   bronchial stenosis, 119
   bronchophony, 118-119
   egophony, 113-116
   noisy breathing, 119

Abnormally transmitted sounds—cont'd
   poor breath sounds/good voice sounds, 119
   whispered pectoriloquy, 117
Acini, 4
Acute epiglottitis, 106, 107f
Acute hoarseness, 108
Adolescent idiopathic scoliosis, 44
Advanced clubbing, 38
Adventitious sounds
   airway obstruction, 111
   bronchial leak squeak, 112-113
   crackles, 88-100. *See also* Crackles.
   croup, 106
   diphtheria, 106-107
   epiglottitis, 106
   hoarseness, 108-110
   inspiratory squawk, 113
   laryngitis, 108
   laryngomalcia, 105-106
   mediastinal crunch, 112
   neoplasms of larynx, 109-110
   pleural friction rub, 111-112
   stridor, 105-108
   vocal cord paralysis, 108-109
   wheezes, 100-105. *See also* Wheezes.
Air hunger, 38, 45
Airway and tissue resistance work, 6f, 7
Airway auscultation, 82-83
Airway obstruction, 11f, 111
Allergic alveolitis, 113
Allergic disorders, 29
Alpha$_1$-antitrypsin deficiency, 15
Alveolar duct, 4, 5f
Alveolar ventilation, 12
Alveoli, 2f, 4, 5f
Anatomy
   chest wall, 4-5
   conducting airways, 1
   terminal respiratory units, 4
   trachea, 2-4
Angular kyphosis, 43

Anterior axillary line, 40, 41f
Aortic pain, 33
Apnea, 45
Asbestosis, 93, 99f, 101f, 103
Assessment. *See* History, Laboratory
    tests, Physical examination.
Asthma, 92
Asthmatic attacks, 29
Atelectasis, 12f, 13, 67t
Atelectasis of left upper lobe, 12f
Auditory tube, 22f
Ausculatory percussion, 54
Auscultation, 64-67

Bacille Calmette-Guérin (BCG), 31
Barrel chest, 42f, 43
BCG, 31
Bell chest piece, 25-26
Binaural hearing, 23f
Biot, Camille, 46
Biot's respiration, 46
Body of sternum, 40f
Bowles chest piece, 25-26
Bradypnea, 45
Breath sound score, 120
Breath sounds. *See* Abnormal breath
    sounds, Normal breath sounds.
Bronchi, 2
Bronchial artery, 5f
Bronchial asthma, 67t
Bronchial breath sounds (tubular), 66
Bronchial breathing, 118
Bronchial leak squeak, 112-113
Bronchial stenosis, 119
Bronchiectasis, 30, 31, 96-97
Bronchitis, 35, 92
Bronchography, 57, 58f
Bronchomotor nerve, 5f
Bronchophony, 118-119
Bronchopulmonary segments, 3f, 4
Bronchoscope, 57
Bronchoscopy, 57
Bronchovesicular breath sounds, 66
Bronchus, 5f
Bullar, J. F., 67

Carbon dioxide tension (PaCO$_2$), 58
Carcinoma of the pyriform fossa, 110
Cardiac dullness, 52f
Cardiac pain, 33
Carlson, C. J., 76
Chapter review, guidelines, 125-131
Chest fluoroscopy, 54
Chest injuries/operations, 31

Chest roentogenogram, 58f
Chest wall
    anatomy, 40f
    examination, 40-45
    lesions, 44-45
    physiology, 4-5
    shape abnormalities, 43-44
Chest wall lesions, 44-45
Chest wall shape abnormalities, 42-44
Cheyne, John, 45
Cheyne-Stokes breathing, 45
Chief complaint, 29
Children
    breath sounds, 73
    stridor, 105-108
Chronic bronchitis, 92
Chronic hoarseness, 108
Chronic laryngitis, 108, 110
Chronic obstructive pulmonary dis-
    ease, 119
Cigarette smoking, 30
Cilia, 33
Clinical tests. *See* Laboratory tests.
Clubbing, 38, 39f
Coarse crackles, 94-96, 121f
Cochlea, 22f
Cochlear nerve, 22f
Compliance work, 6f, 7
Compressive atelectasis, 13
Computerized axial tomography, 55
Conducting airways, 1
Congenital atelectasis, 13
Congenital narrowing of larynx, 107,
    108f
Congenital stridor, 105
Consolidation, 14f, 15, 67t
Corynebacterium diphtheriae, 106
Costal angle, 40f
Costal margin, 40f
Costochondral junctions, 40f
Costochondral pain, 32
Cough, 33-34
Cough syncope, 34
Crackle simulator, 91f
Crackles, 88-100
    bronchiectasis, 96-97
    coarse, 94-96
    early inspiratory, 91, 92f
    fine, 94-96
    incidence/types, 97t, 98f, 99f, 101f
    late inspiratory, 92, 93f
    obstructive disease, in, 91-92
    posturally induced, 99
    restrictive disease, in, 92-94